For Sylvia, my dear
new friend + neighbor ~
fellow writer -

may your journeys down
our beach, to our beach,
always be healing
                Truly,
                Karen

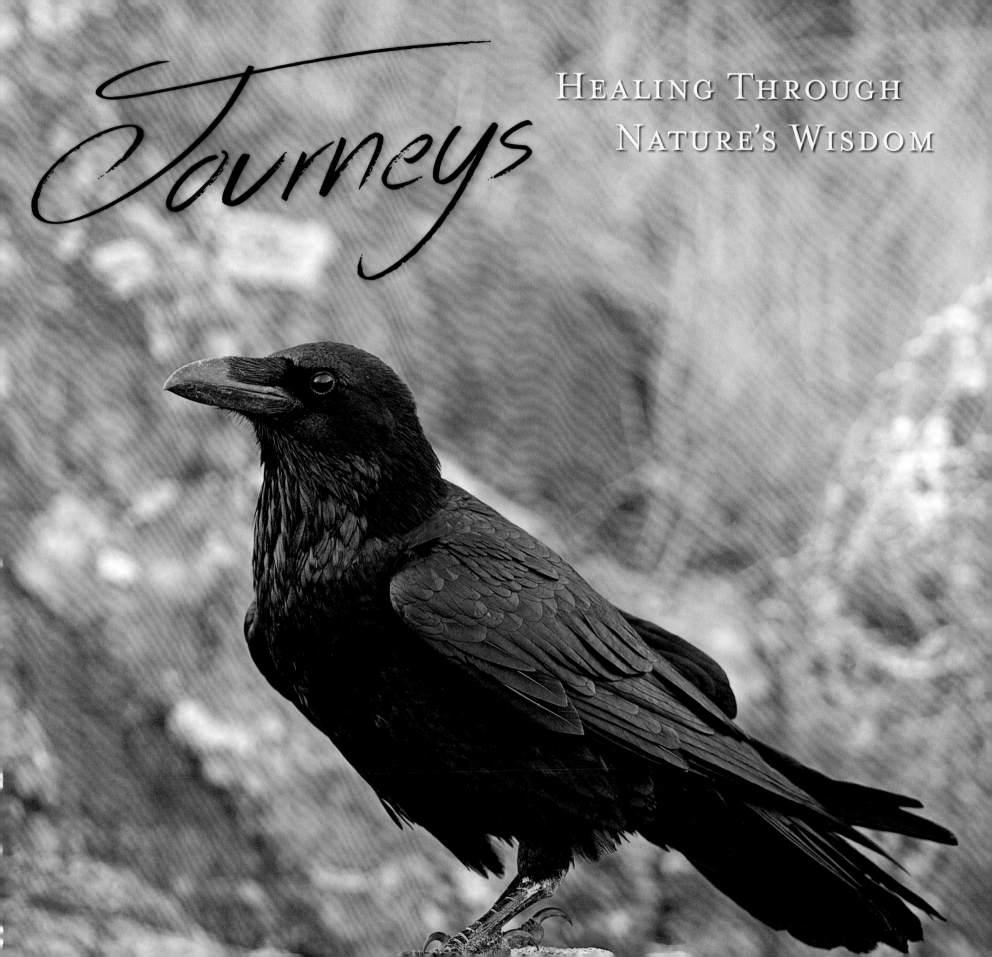

Journeys

Healing Through Nature's Wisdom

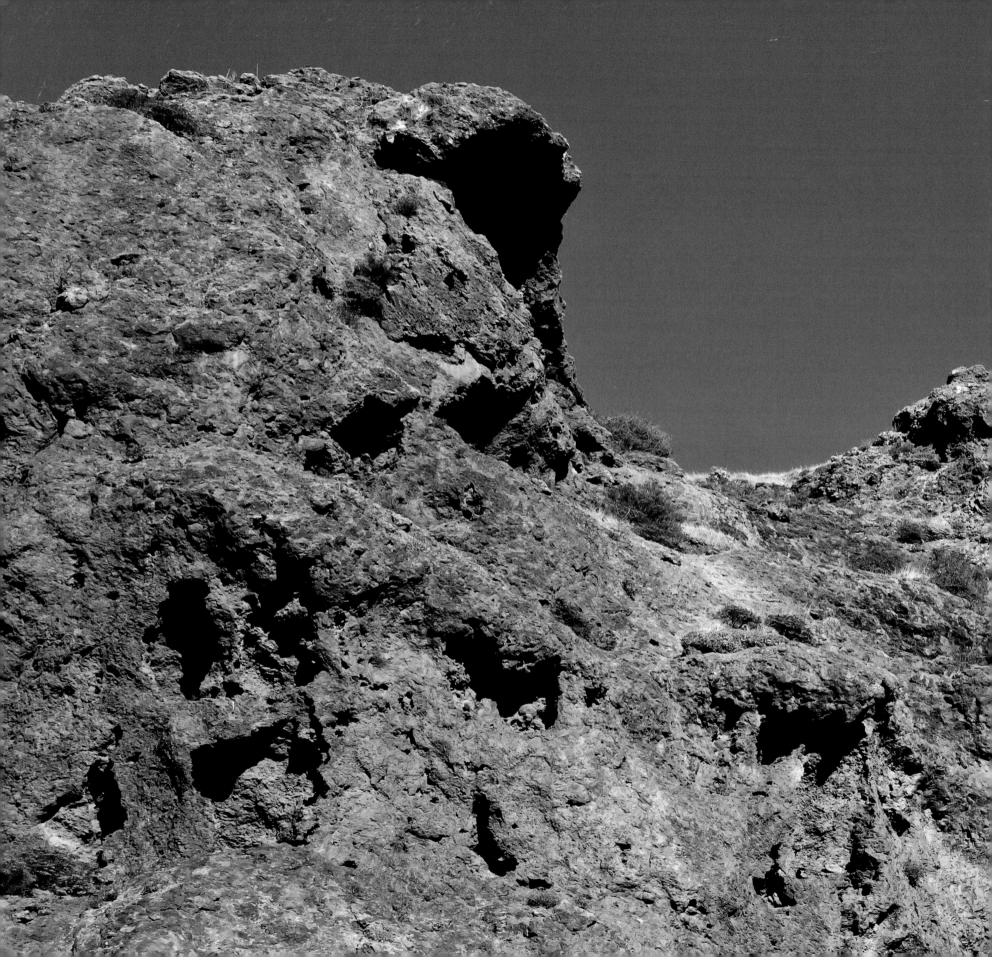

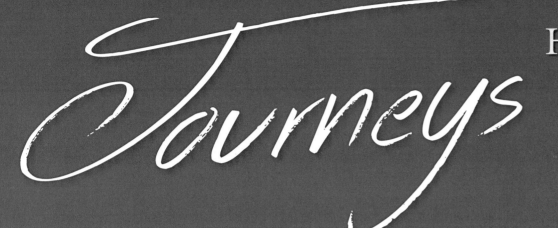

Journeys

HEALING THROUGH NATURE'S WISDOM

ESSAYS BY KAREN ROBERTS
AND DANA SIMPSON

PHOTOGRAPHY BY TIM HAUF

Journeys: Healing through Nature's Wisdom

Essays by Karen Roberts and Dana Simpson
Photography by Tim Hauf

Published by Tim Hauf Photography, P.O. Box 1241, Kingston, WA 98346, USA.

Copyright © 2015 Tim Hauf Photography

Library of Congress Control Number: 2014914020

ISBN: 978-0-9788219-7-5

Website: www.timhaufphotography.com
www.healingthroughnatureswisdom.com

Email: timhauf@hotmail.com or tim@healingthroughnatureswisdom.com

Author Contacts
Karen Roberts: karen@healingthroughnatureswisdom.com
Dana Simpson: dana@healingthroughnatureswisdom.com

Copy editor: Linda Davis ldavis@writtenword.net

Content editor: Douglas Glenn Clark dgwrite@gmail.com

Proofreader: Courtney Hlebo courtneyhlebo@gmail.com

Publicist: Gail Kearns gail@topressandbeyond.com

Printed and bound in Manitoba, Canada

First printing: February 2015

The secret of health for both mind and body is not to mourn for the past, not to worry about the future, but to live in the present moment wisely and earnestly.

—BUDDHA

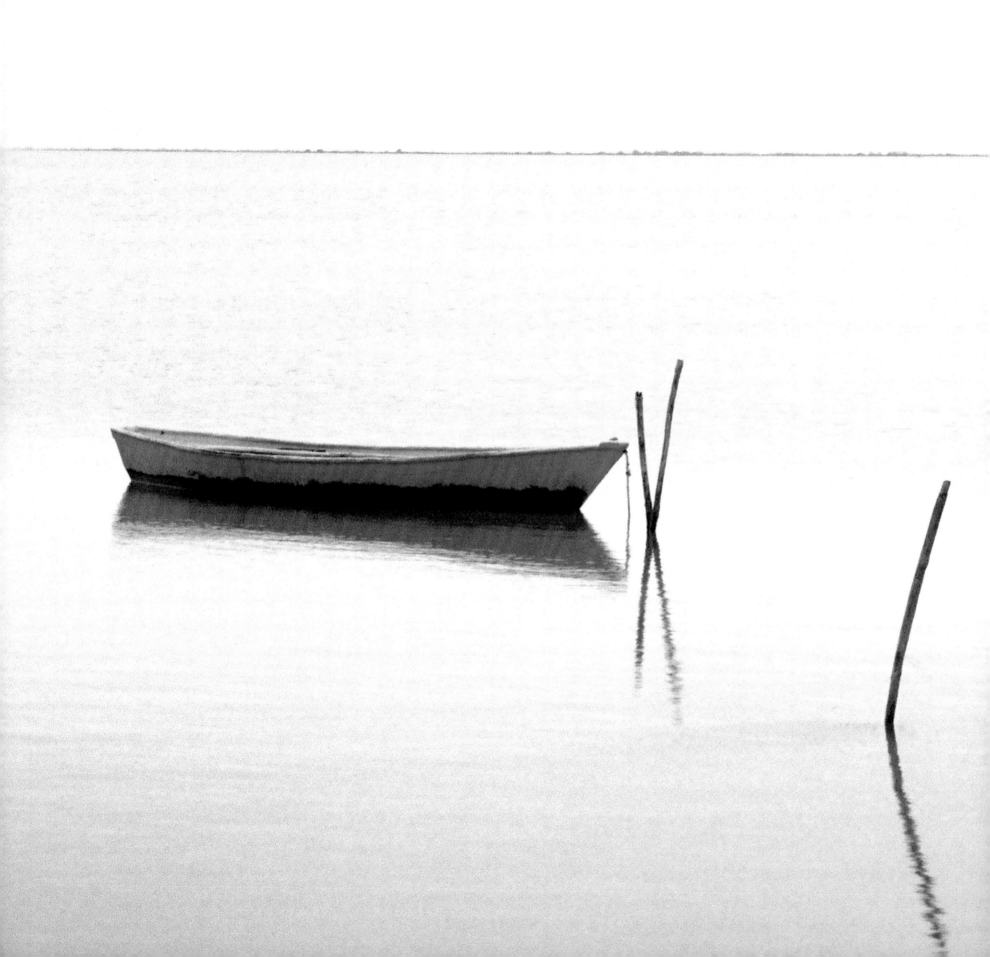

Table of Contents

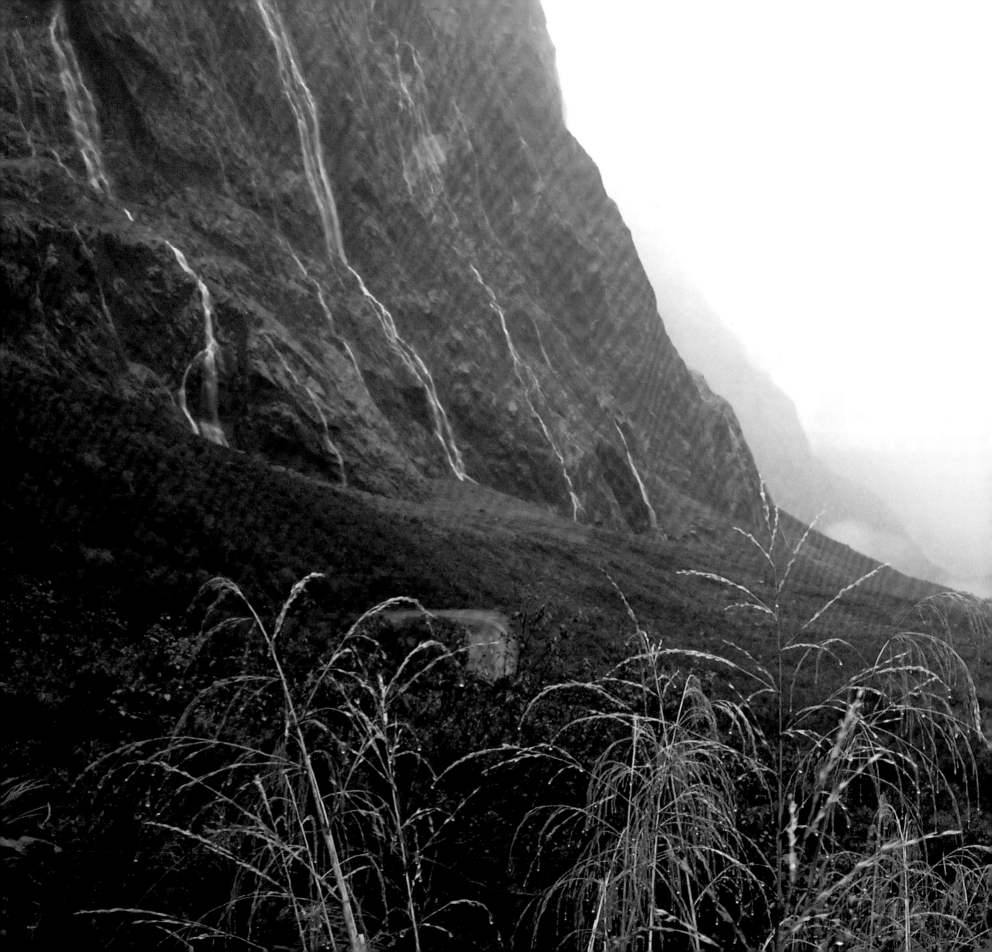

Introduction

Our personal essays herein were written to give you hope if you are challenged by physical limitations or if, like us, you suffer from a condition doctors can't diagnose or resolve. Incurable illness can overwhelm us with feelings of fear and vulnerability, replacing confidence and the successes of earlier times. Multiple sclerosis and Lyme disease are our afflictions. Whatever yours may be, we hope these healing journeys inspire you.

Our exploration of what is possible is not meant to challenge, but to encourage. The medical practices of the Western world may be our first recourse, but not our last. Leaving the sickbed and bedroom behind are huge first steps. If you do not trust your body to do it alone, we hope to walk beside you. The bravery to say "maybe" to new horizons is huge because following an impulse often feels awkward, even impossible. Discovering possibilities and embracing dreams are personal pursuits that can lead to unexpected outcomes and victories.

New horizons require new perspectives—we needed to find freedom first, a separation from past conditioning and demands that our schooling, our families, and our society had given us. Freedom from the striving that drove our early years. When we no longer demanded of ourselves but let nature direct us, we found healing paths.

We restarted our lives without expectations. Going outside, experiencing nature as a marvelous gift was our medicine. Birdsong and gentle breezes replaced sadness and fear. Observing the life of tide pools and the curiosity of a camera lens brought us back to a state of well-being and wonder.

Clinical studies have shown the benefits of meditation and relaxation when healing. Our travels essentially provided both—plus the exhilarating sense of discovery.

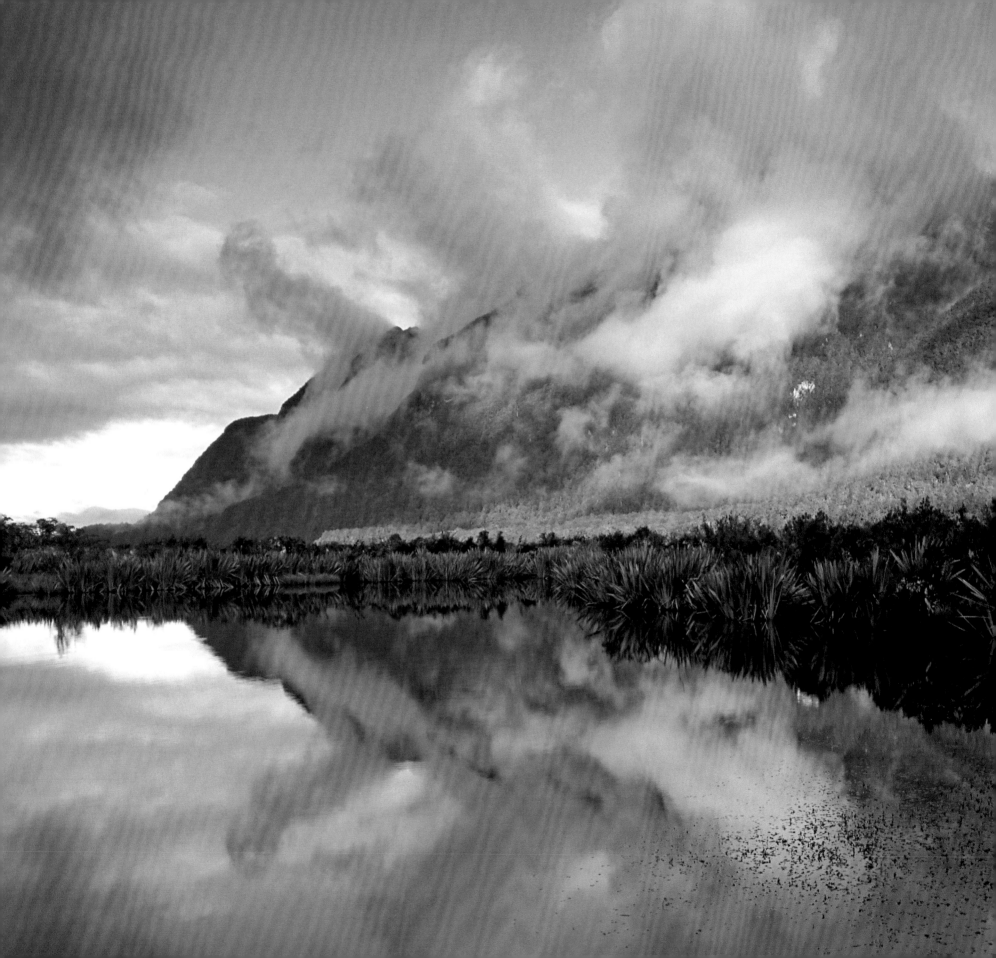

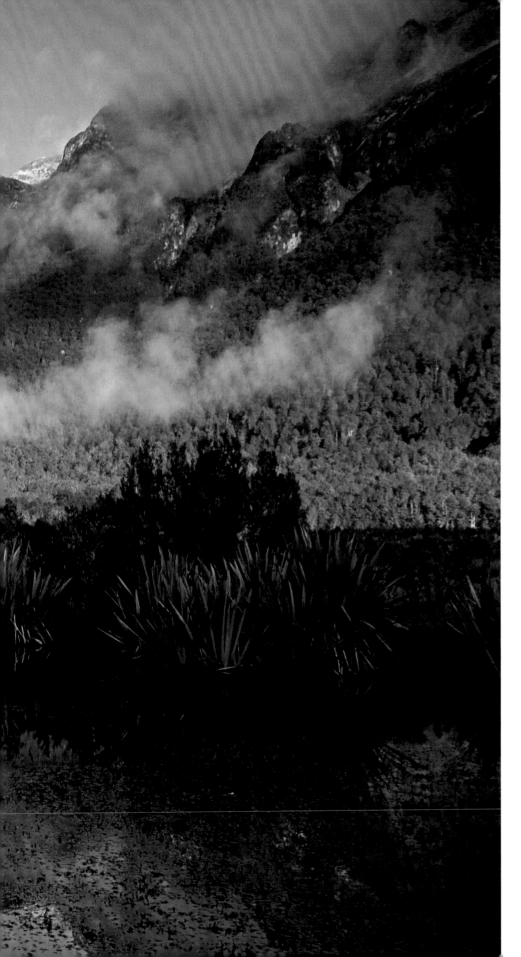

Shear Harmony
New Zealand

Maybe I could. Picking up a camera to capture special places might be something permitted in spite of MS. And so I began, enjoying the mystery of light, the magic of color as the sun dropped in the sky. Landscapes pulled me away. I found a teacher, Tim Hauf, professional photographer, who guided me to experiment with different lenses, different apertures, to use the natural light. Take time to frame the image: color interest in foreground, balanced scene behind. Photography could be slow, methodical, and surprisingly possible.

Empowered by my Nikon and Tim's encouragement, we went on a photo journey to New Zealand. He had been there many times, once even led a photography group. So we were off, but nothing prepared me for the "land down under."

Thousands of sheep cover the hillsides like an endless plain of gentle waves, so synchronized in their movement that the silky animals are barely perceptible. They are the landscape in New Zealand, and I fell in love with them. They reminded me of my own childhood blanket decorated with pastoral scenes that included these peaceful animals. In a psychology class I once took, I learned that young monkeys reach for sheepskin metal mommies before food, showing their need for physical touch over life-sustaining gruel. As I gazed at these sheep now, my body felt caressed by their reassuring softness.

Driving south on the South Island, I wondered if we were heading for the end of the earth, as we seemed to pass forever through empty lands, except for the sheep. In the distance, there were snowy peaks, but here below, only grassy hills and a spaciousness I'd never known. As we slowly made our way onward, a sense of timelessness took over, a separation from the busy world of before. The vastness invited opening, a freedom to be someone new, in my case a photographer.

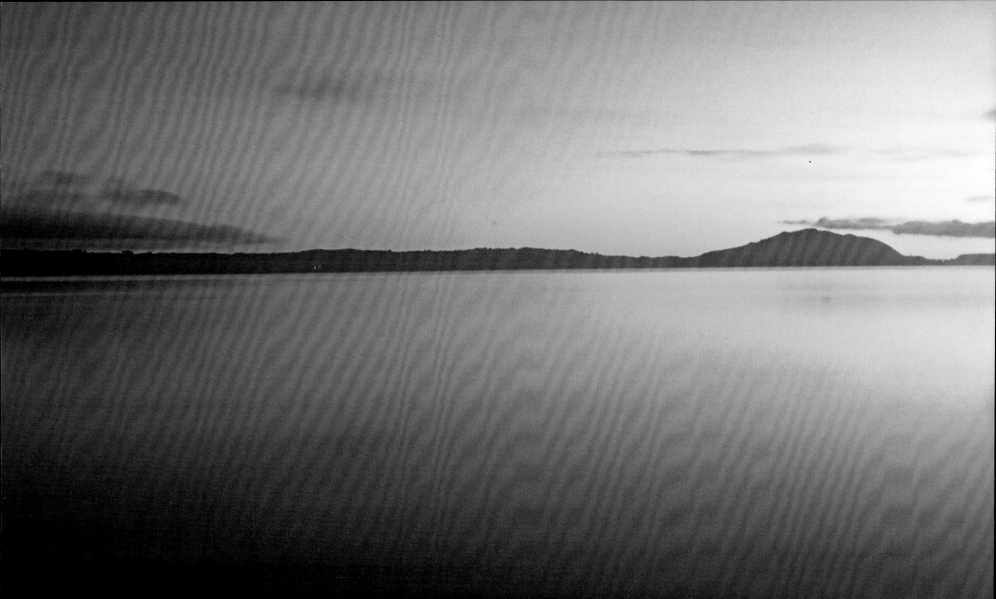

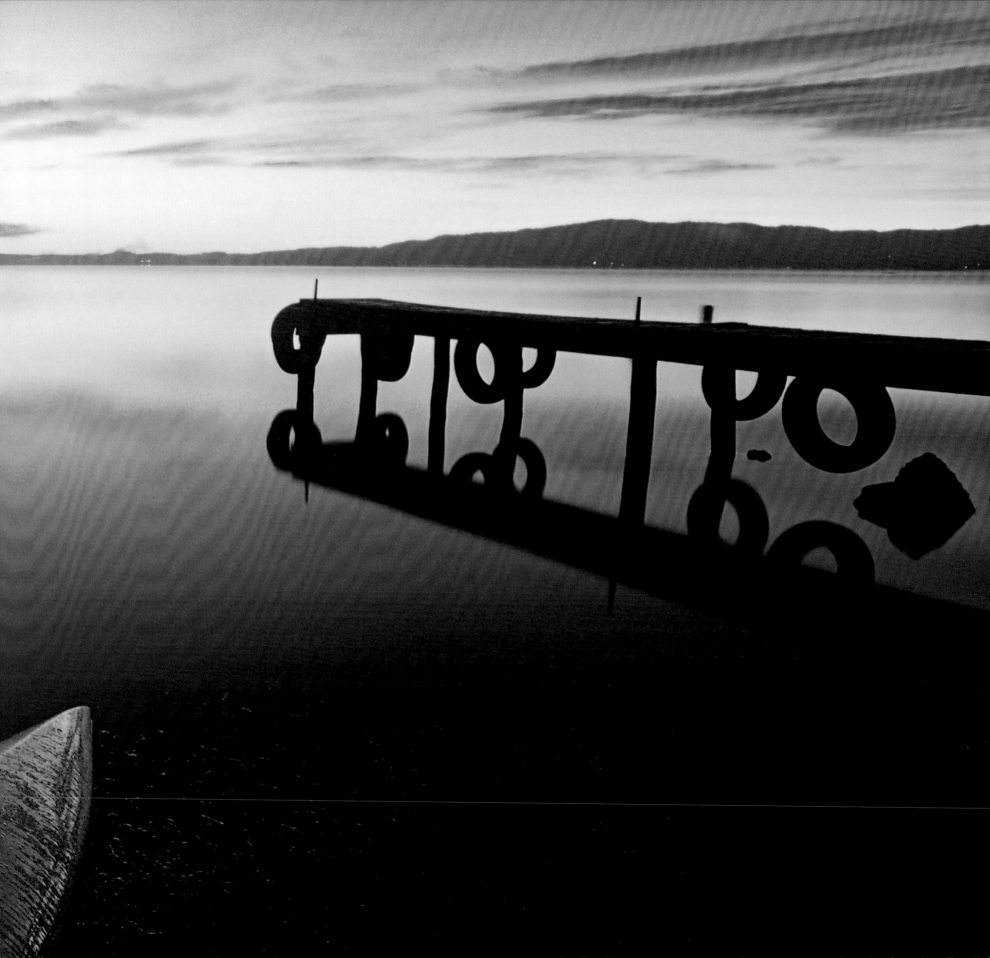

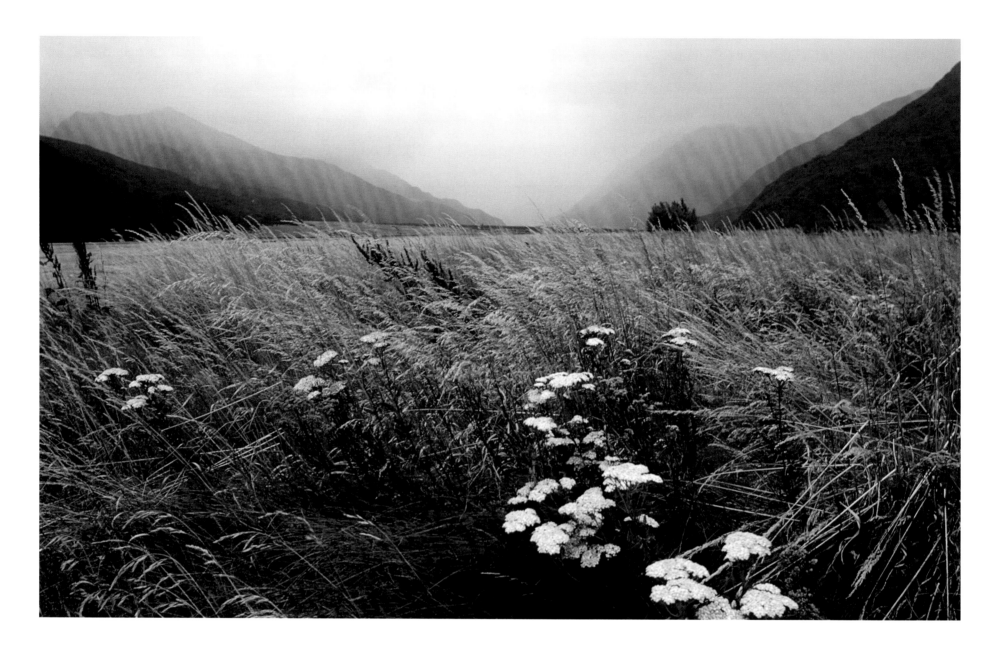

I reflected on a year in my youth when I raised a lamb through the National 4-H program. I was healthy then and undaunted by the daily tasks of feeding and walking, cleaning pen and animal alike. I had neither gratitude for the body that did these things nor a sense of harmony in the daily rituals. Decades later, when carrying buckets or raking the earth weren't possible, I searched for a path that would make me whole again. If no medicines were available to cure me, then what? I remembered all the care I had given my sheep, and the 4-H pledge of giving my head, heart, hands, health in service to my community. I was a devoted and disciplined caregiver. Now, I needed to care for myself.

Western medicine provided a diagnosis, but no direction on how to live with my condition. I pulled into myself. I read and meditated. The answer I received was to go outside, to ask the plants and trees, the birds and small beings. In nature, I discovered calmness and sweetness, rhythms of life that included me without requiring any action. Most of my life, I had pushed myself to extraordinary lengths. I now discovered two more values to add to my pledge: hope and help. With hope, I never stopped believing I would find a way back to a stronger body, and accepting help opened me to guidance. I followed my friend with a camera across the sea and land to the farthest post on a foreign continent.

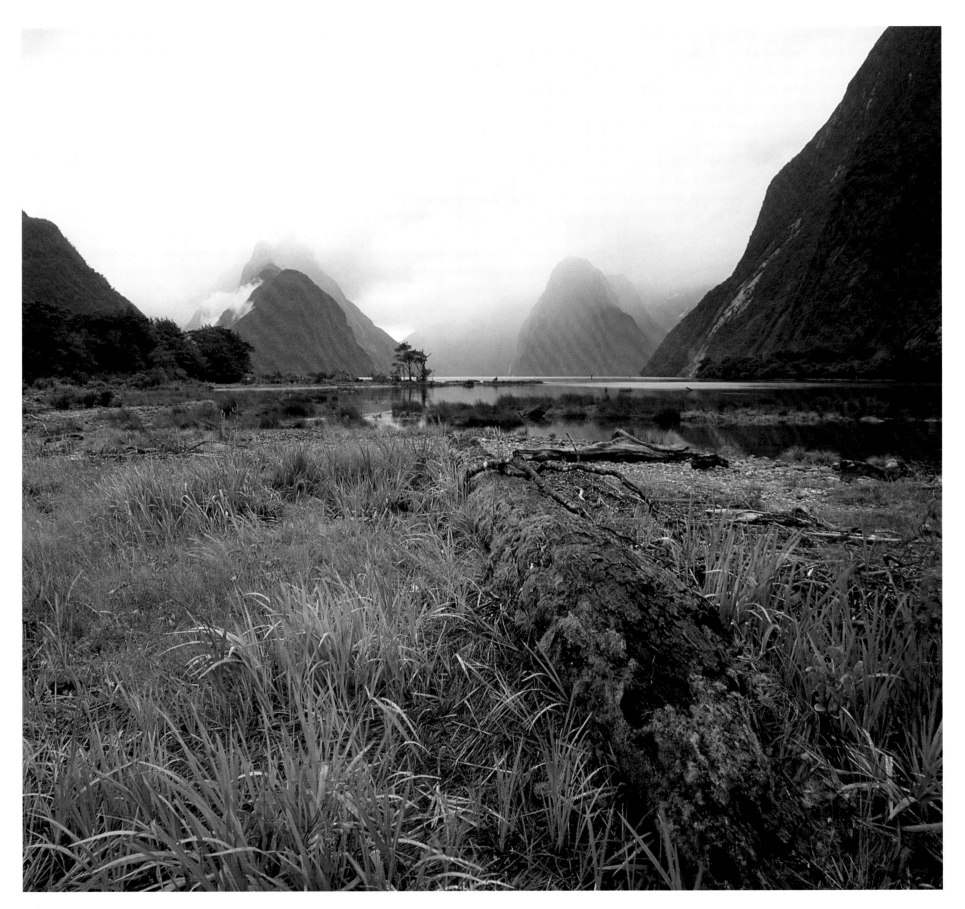

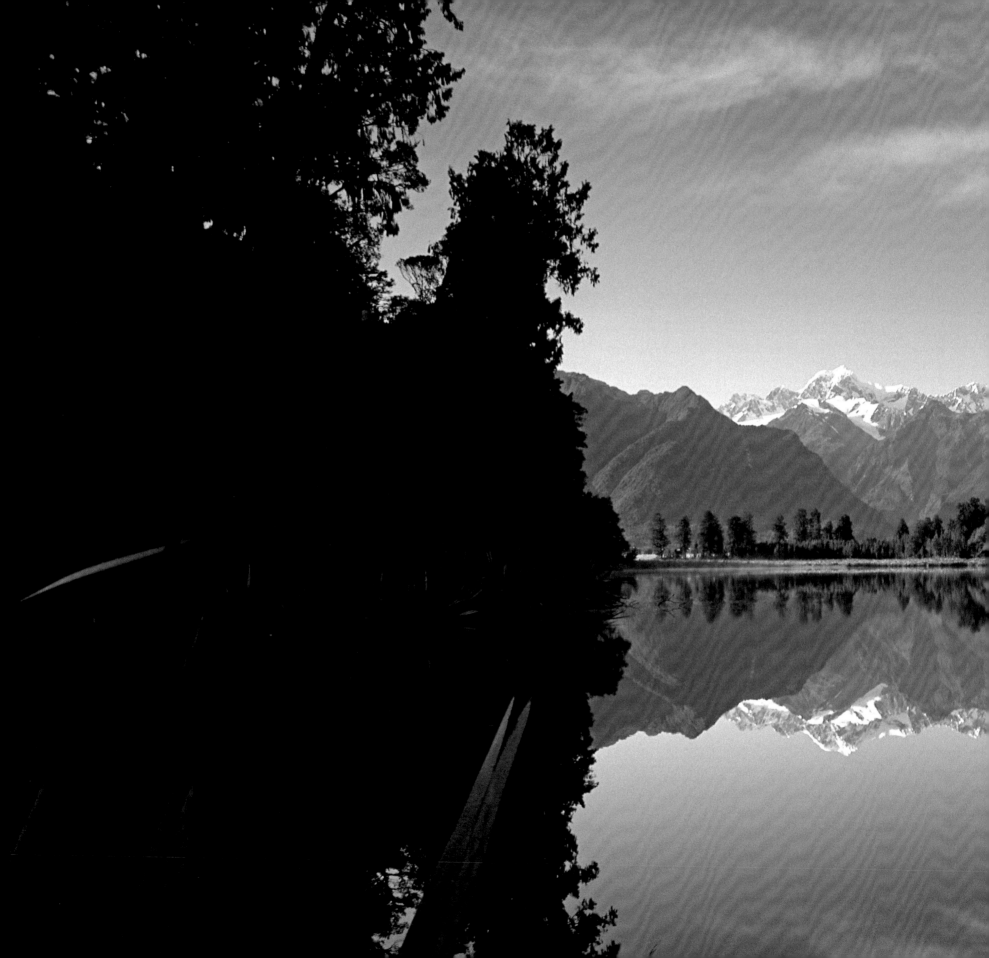

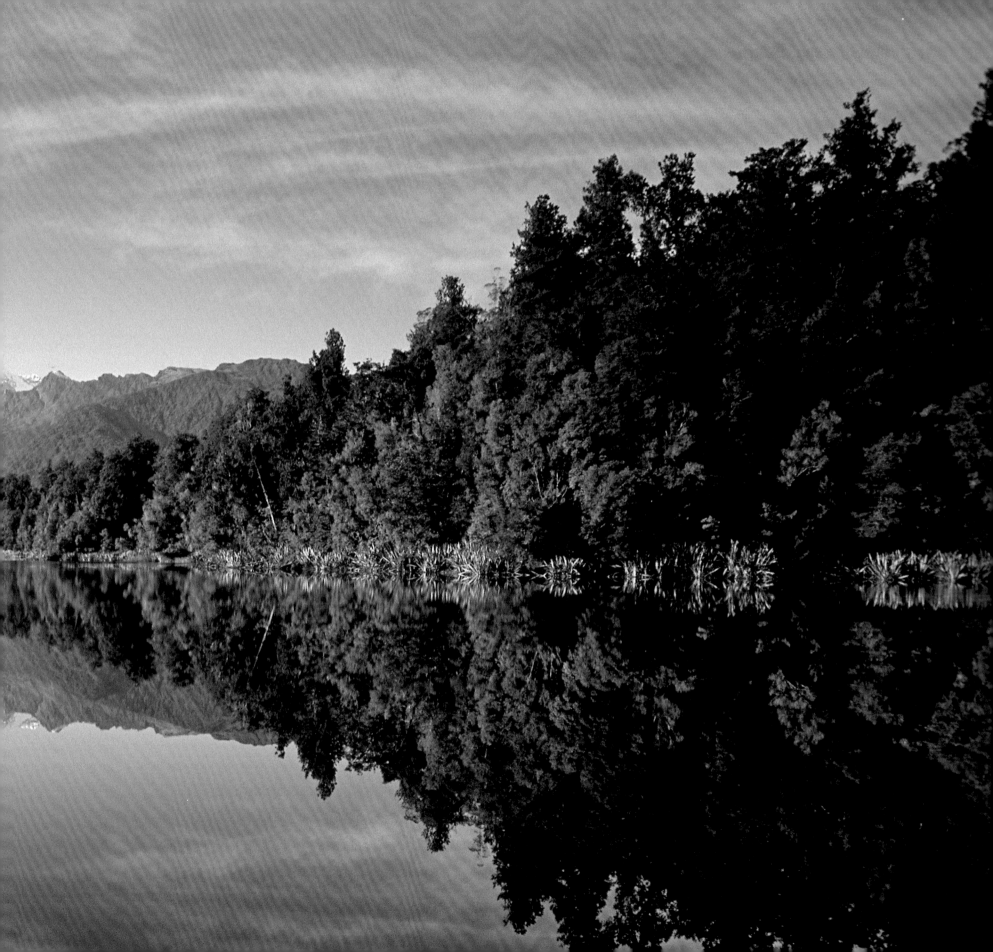

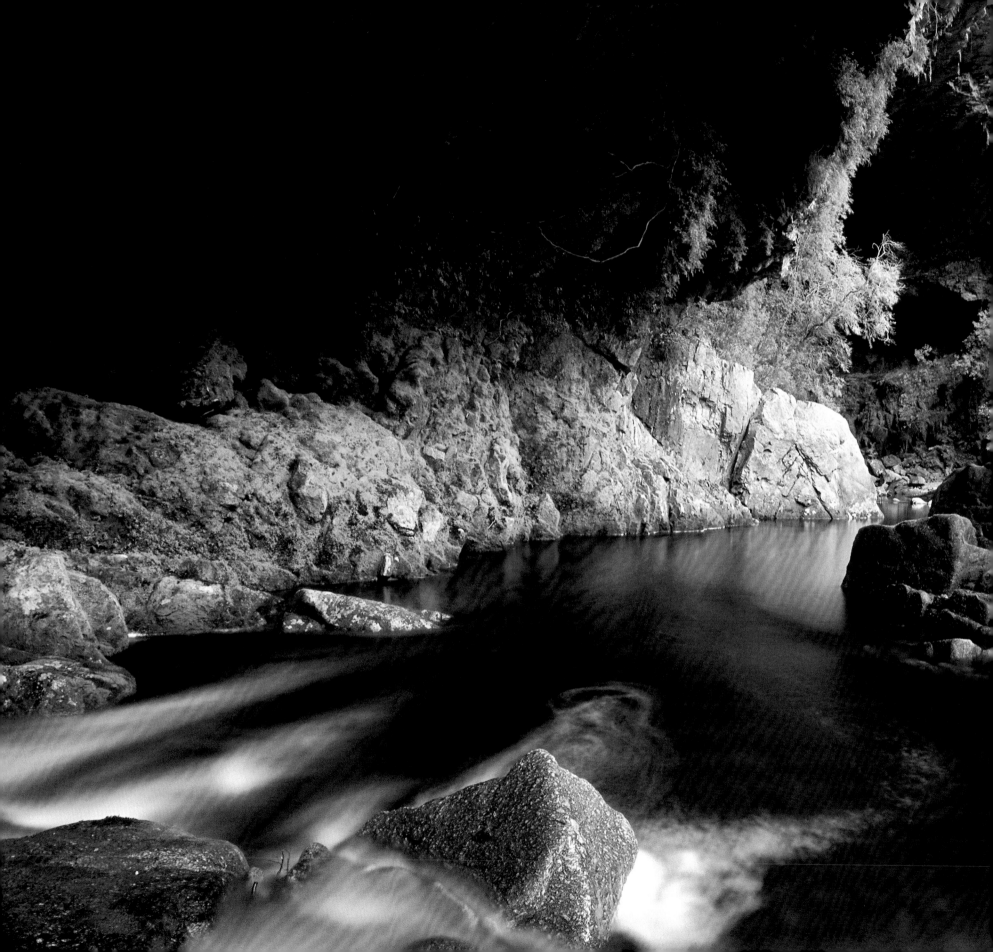

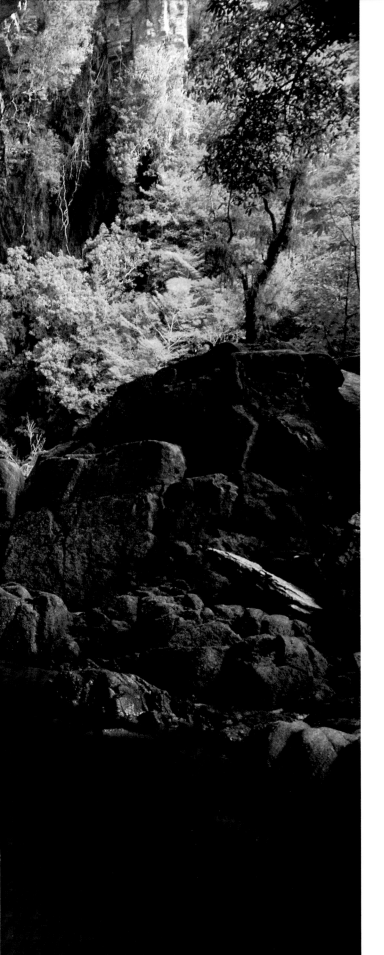

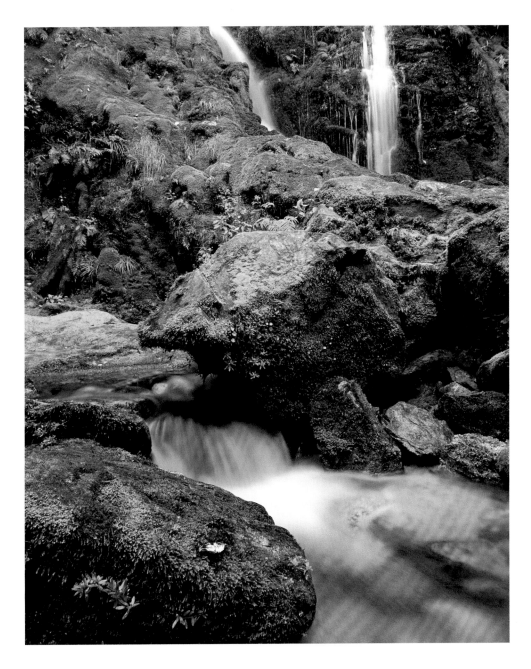

Arthur's Pass is an old sheep station with a multitude of paths through high regions of history, both natural and man-made. When news of a local shearing reached us, we followed our curiosity to watch this traditional custom. Initially, we saw a violent scene. Two hefty men, shirtsleeves rolled, worked in rapid unison: One man tossed the heavy sheep on their sides, pinning them down on the cement floor, while the other approached with shears in hand. The entire pelt was removed in three or four pieces before the animal was released, shaking as she rose and bolted to rejoin her mates. We later learned these same men, brothers, returned every season to shear these sheep who endured the brief onslaught without struggle or complaint.

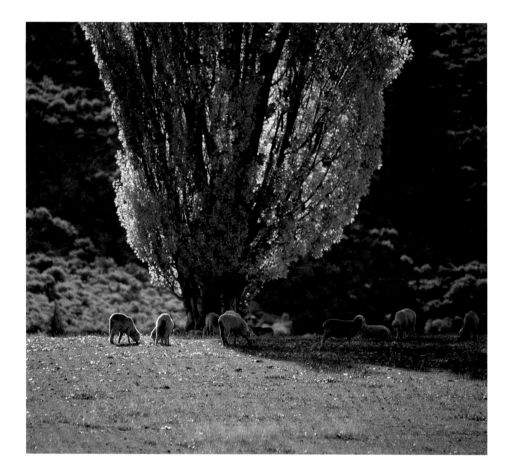

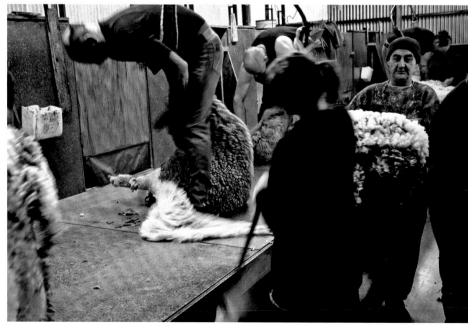

That morning we observed a special harmony between human and animal: man removing a heavy unwanted coat of fur, animal succumbing, trusting. The men worked with such quiet and quick movements that it was like a symphony. The men would perhaps shear another sixty to eighty sheep by nightfall. We emerged from the shed wordlessly, Tim having grown up on a farm in North Dakota, I in an urban American city. It was a gift to observe an ancient ritual, as most sheep shearers around the world have given up scissors for mechanized modern ways.

At first my own feelings of vulnerability made me empathize with the sheep because I feared they might feel assaulted. Yet the comforting, reassuring manner of the shearing team put the animals at ease. I was relieved to watch them scamper away unharmed and free of a heavy coat of fur.

This place opened me to a space of balance, and watching these men with the sheep showed me an active harmony. My physical being released long-held tensions. I took a deep breath of country air and knew a smile would return whenever I thought of the miracle of care and understanding I had watched.

The dogs yelped happily, and we silently said our thanks.

—Karen

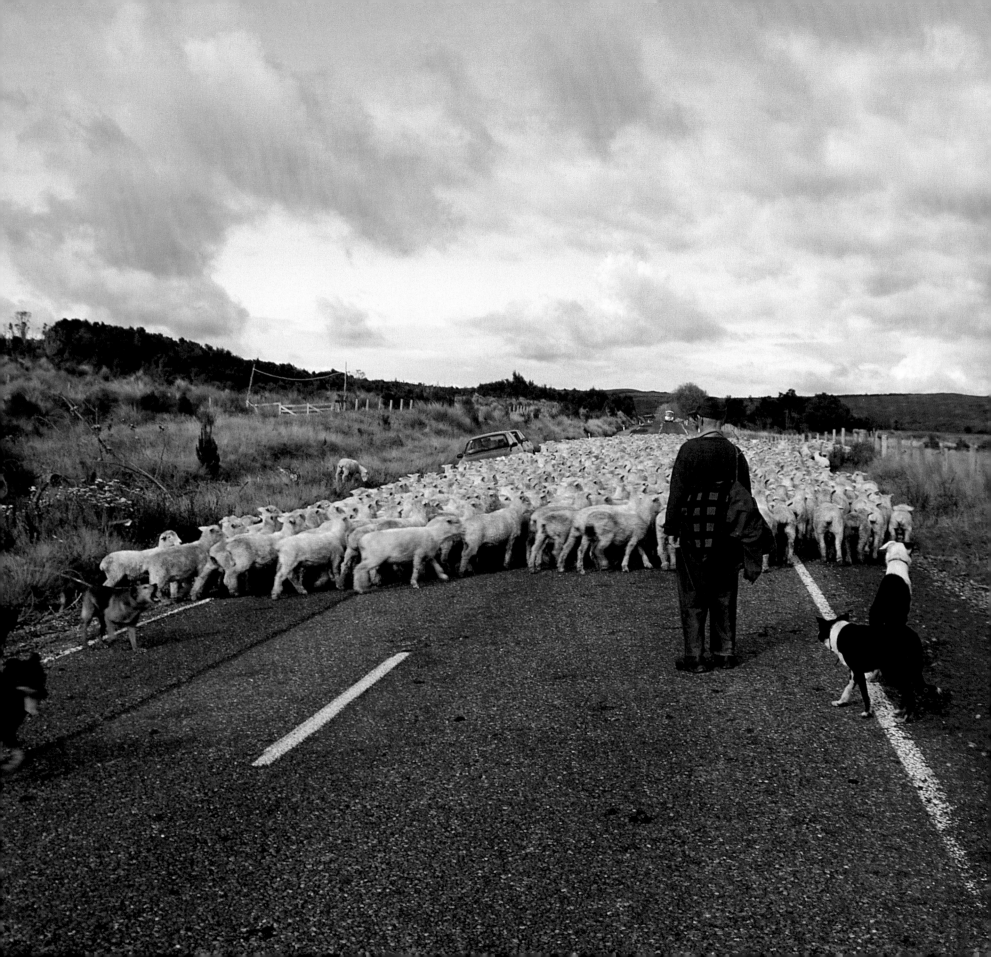

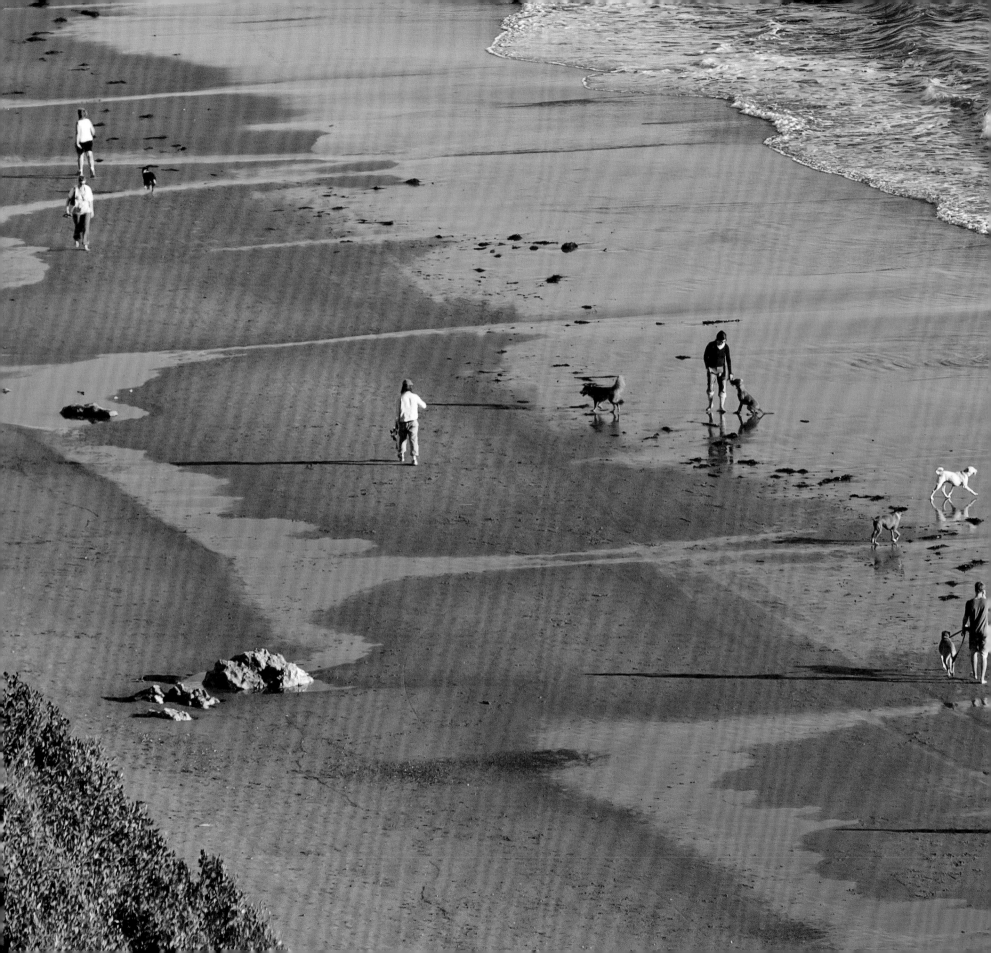

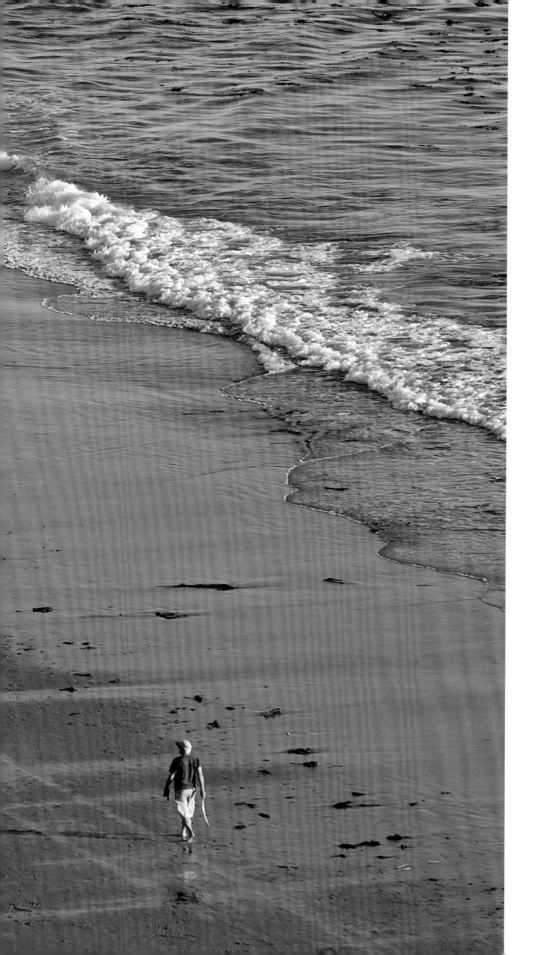

Sand and Soil

Santa Barbara, California

A leg injury hamstrung me for nearly a decade. The chronic pain led me through many doors; it manifested questions about trust, balance, pattern, fear, control, truth. I confronted the paralysis of inaction before I realized how to open myself to the experience of embodiment, of the physical presence of the body. Accepting my condition and making choices in response to pain and discomfort were completely new to me. My tendency had been to "endure" and "overcome," when in fact reassessment and readjustment were required. I needed to learn how to restore a very depleted body. I began reading and learning about disease and health. I then took a step outside and found the wild ones, and the wildness within. I believe wellness is a manifestation we each carry that is constantly changing. Our bodies are not meant to feel the same each moment. They communicate; you can listen.

It may have been despair that drove me to the edge of the seashore, but I believe there was a deeper need to feel a rhythm. The tide pulled in debris, deposited shells, filled in footsteps. I pounded the sand of Hendry's Beach in Santa Barbara, California, for most of a summer. I dragged my body to the farthest cove, where I felt the possibility of my own regeneration. In the beginning, I only seemed able to find the suffering. Before my eyes appeared sea birds with missing feet, broken legs, dragging wings. I must have met every harmed, malformed little animal in that entire stretch. I began to ask myself how I could help. This pivotal question shifted me towards action. I tried to protect the injured birds from frisky dogs, and I filled a bag with trash each day I returned to explore.

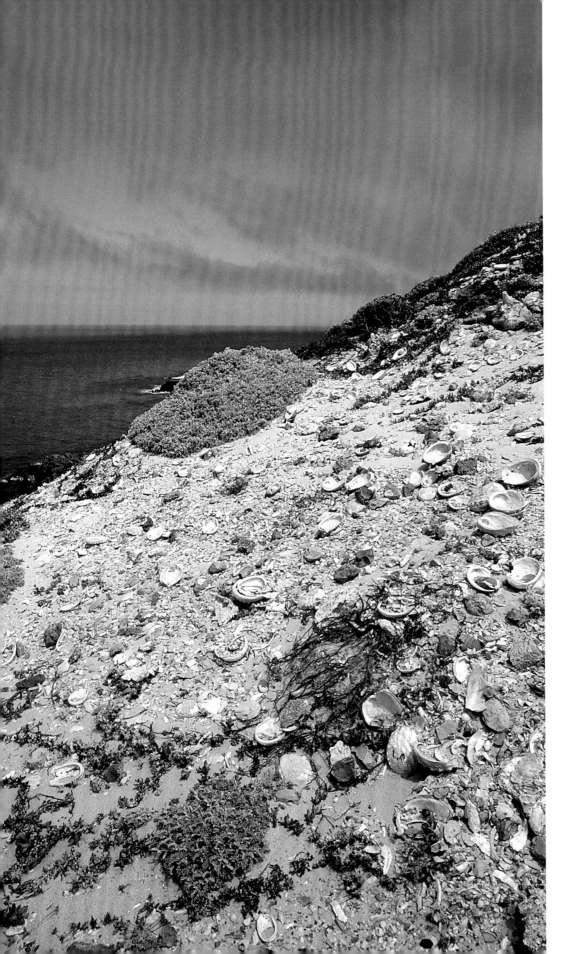

My hands started to reach out to the rocks and shells. Something draws us to select a shell—spiraling into infinity, painted by tumbling waves and burrowing sea creatures. I collected vessels and released them in the current. As I admired them, I began to acknowledge the great mystery and diversity of living forms. The unity that connects us also supports our uniqueness. The smooth, tumbled stones were engraved with pictograms from their travels. These rocks and shells were encouraging, like messages in a bottle sent by a castaway. From a distant shore, they helped me believe in myself. There were days when I gathered rocks with holes, and others that resembled hearts.

Out of the heart shape created by the two halves of a mussel shell, I saw wings. Holding the delicate "shell wings" one afternoon, I contemplated the rigid exoskeleton—the shellfish's structure and strength revealed in this enduring object. What are wings? Symbols of protection, discovery, tenderness, guidance, and flight. There is a connection deeper than structural similarity between wings, and hearts, and lungs. Wings: gentle movement, shifting place, expansive vision. Heart: beat of life, compassion. Lungs: breath of life. I thought of the love that makes us fly. Such ideas made me think it might be time to leave the shore for higher ground.

Standing in dry creek beds, I imagined the force that brought rocks tumbling down mountain slopes to rest before me. Balance had overcome movement. I sensed the surge of water running past, sculpting and chiseling, exposing surface, creating form, the course once traveled by each massive stone revealed in dramatic grooves across its face. I considered my own place in this grand continuum. My walks turned to gardens where I found I stepped more lightly. When did I stop listening to my own body and ignore the symptoms of pain? Will I do it again?

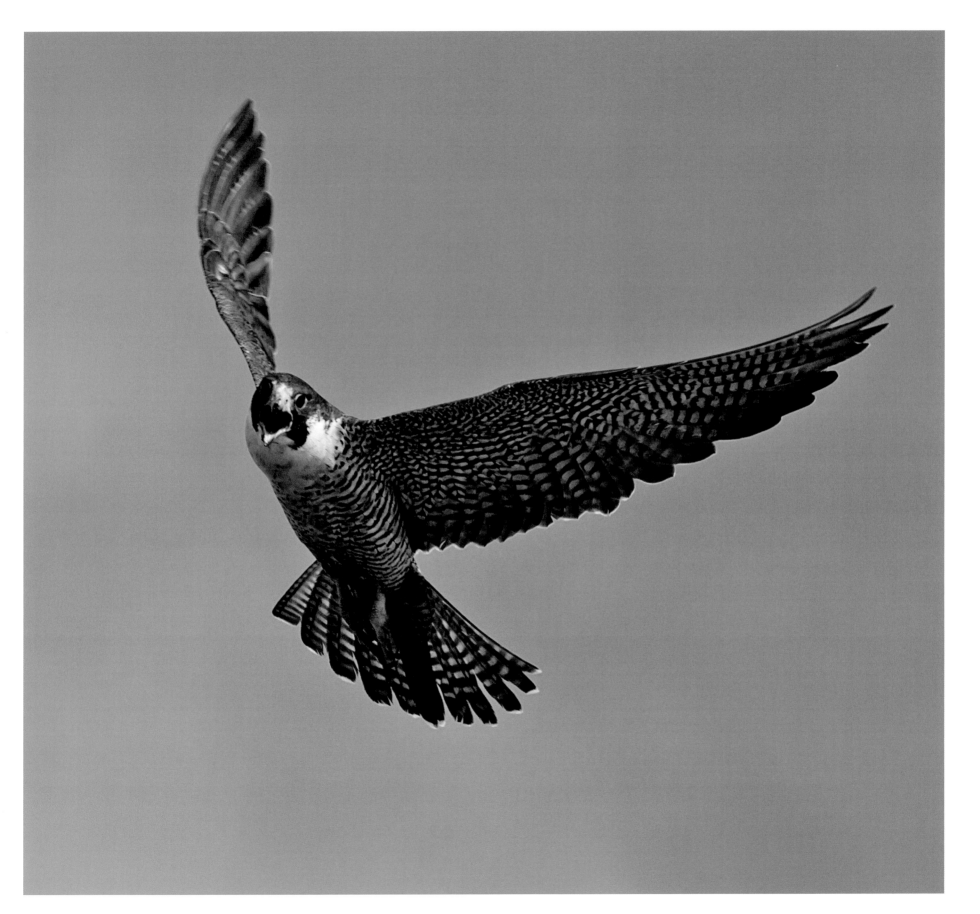

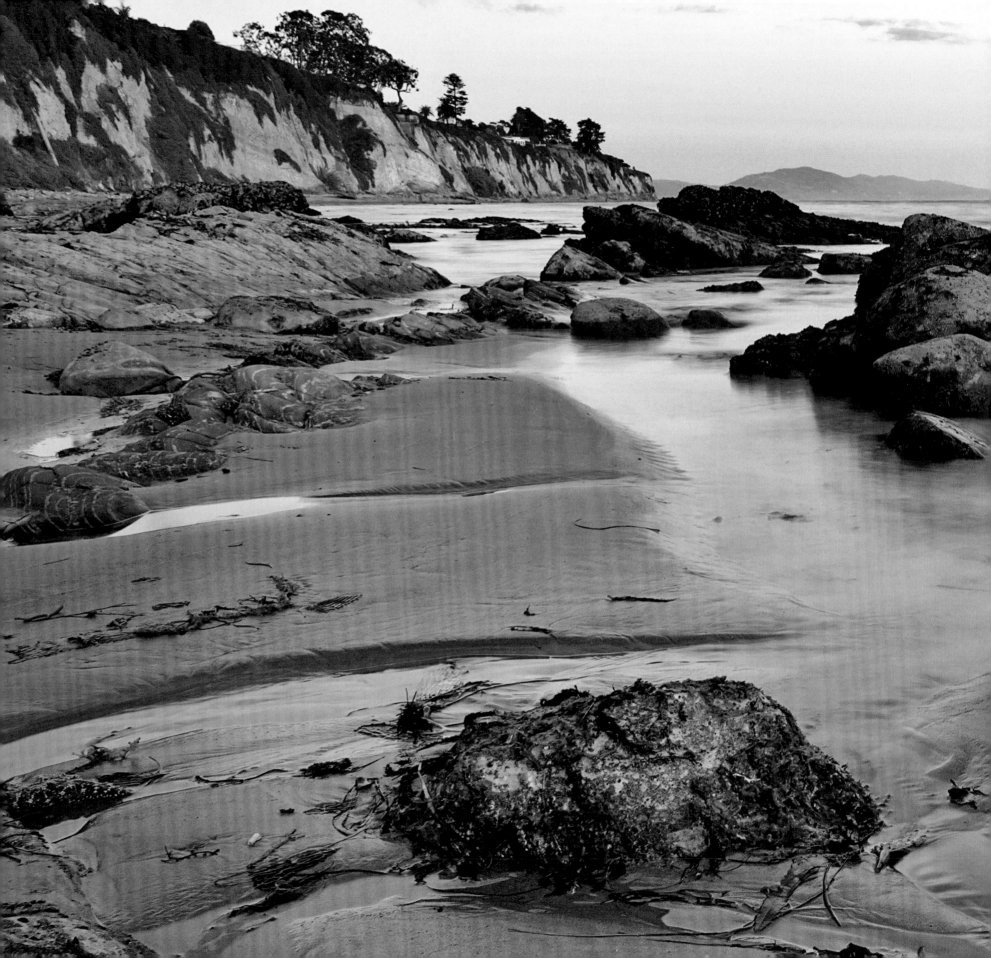

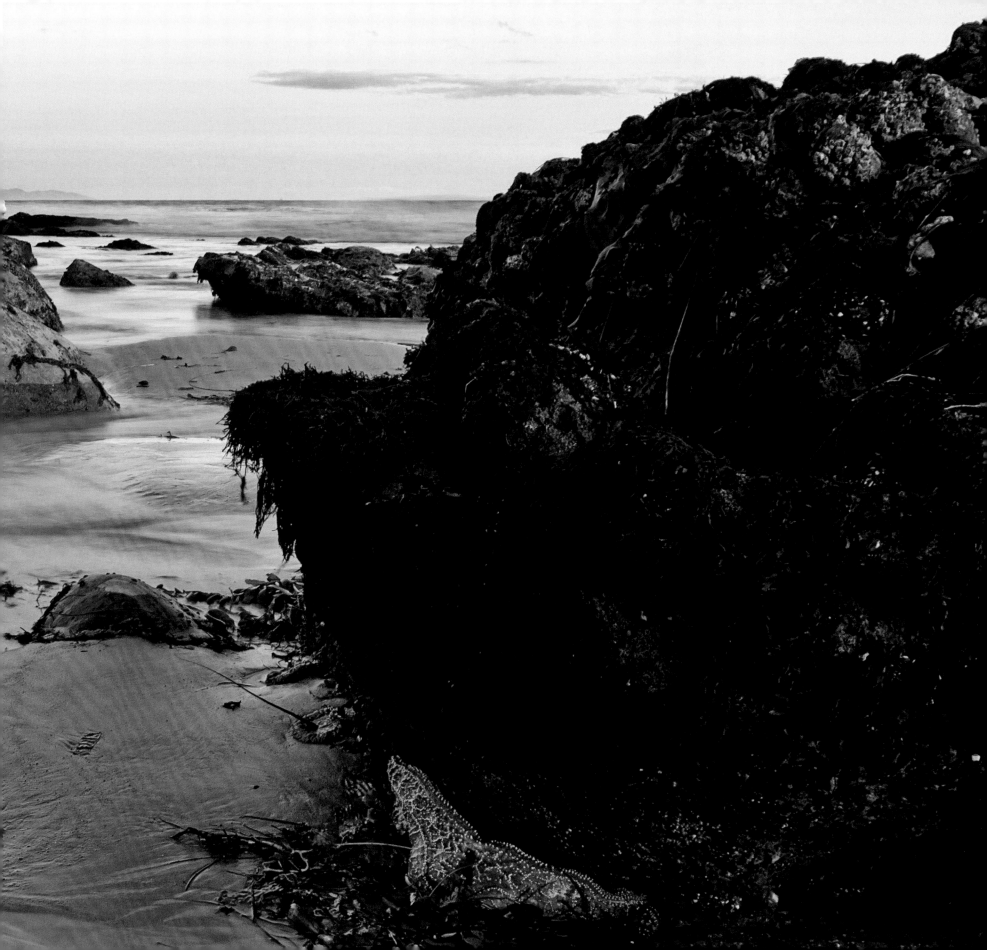

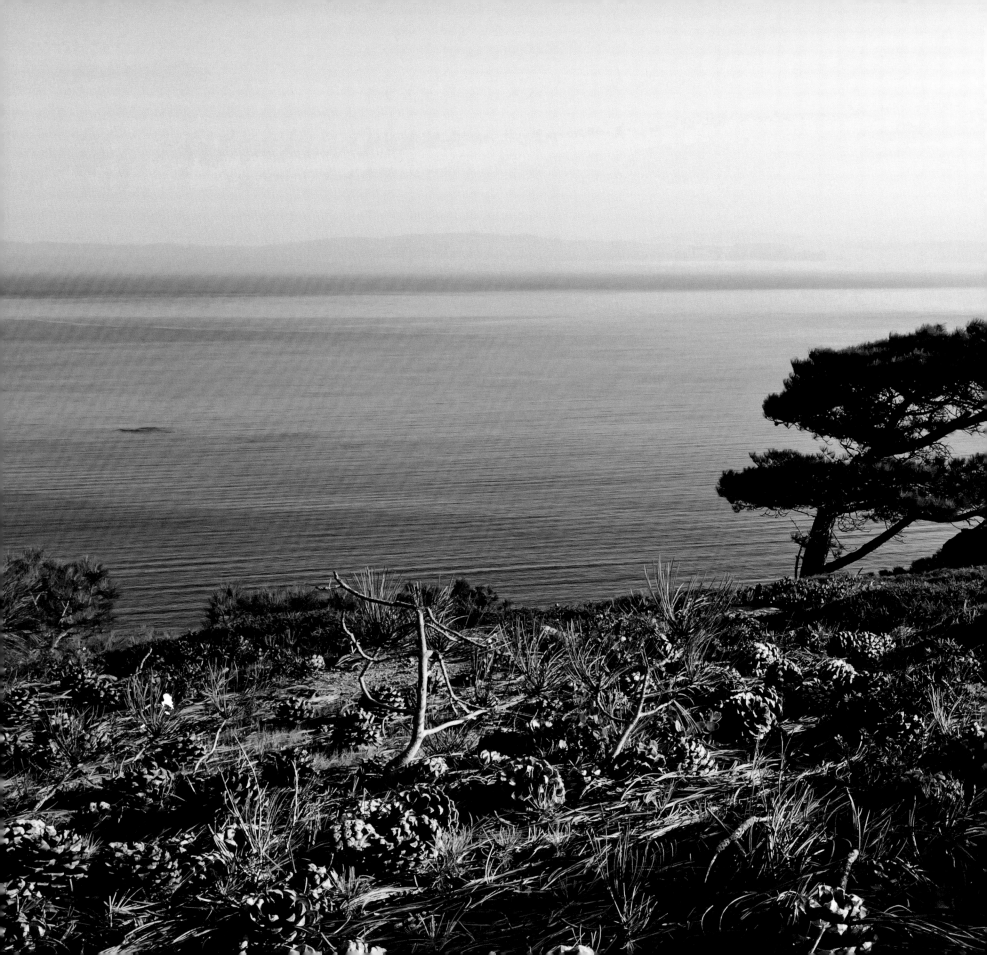

Turning a pinecone in my hand to receive a dusting of pollen or taking in the fragrance of a flower, I let my senses guide me. Opening to these experiences revealed how pain had stagnated my perceptions. With the flower of a trumpet vine in hand, I considered how air transforms into sound as it journeys through this instrument. I began to think about my own voice. Why does pain take away our voice? This remarkable ability to sense we are not well is an opportunity for us to realize how our body communicates. To heal is to allow the integration of mind and body once again.

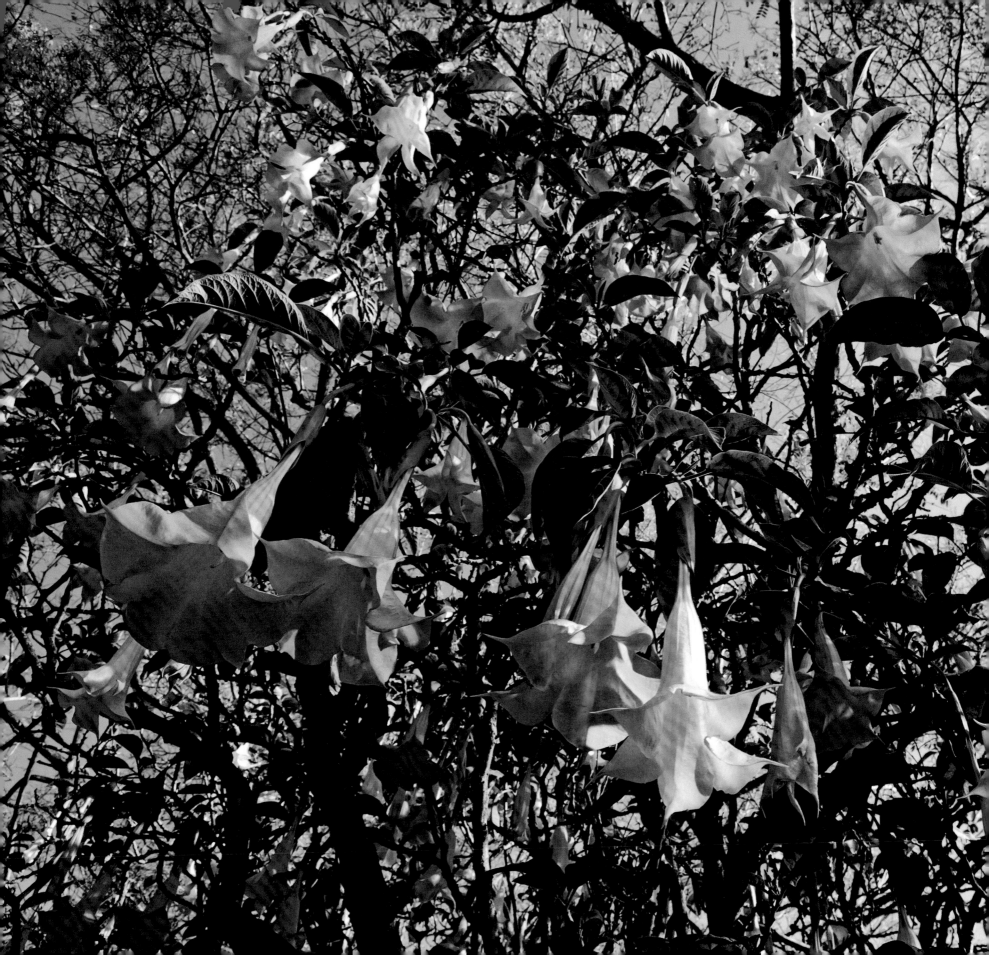

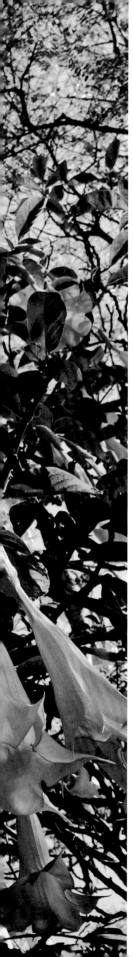

I rested in the grass at Alice Keck Park Memorial Gardens, a few blocks west of downtown Santa Barbara, and got lost in my twitching leg muscles. I surrendered to something both corporeal and cosmic, and thought about how forgiving the body is, how it is resistant when necessary, or supple and flexible when warranted. I took off my shoes and circled the sundial that is embedded in a floor of stones. In my socks, I practiced walking, shifting weight from right foot to left. Once the heel has contact with the ground, the other foot may rise. In the center of this park, I regained my own walk.

I came upon a female turtle that had wandered from the large pond. A gardener was nearby, and I alerted him. I asked if she was sick. He told me she was laying her eggs. I asked why she had traveled so far from the pond. "The pressures of overpopulation," he said. She was searching for a new pond. Instinct was attempting to ensure survival of the next generation. The turtle reminded me that being alone only really matters when we are searching for ways to serve life. I had been spending too much time examining my condition and needed to end my isolation. Thus began my six-month apprenticeship with the park's master gardener.

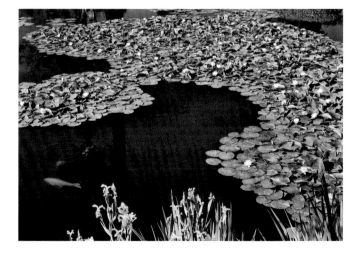

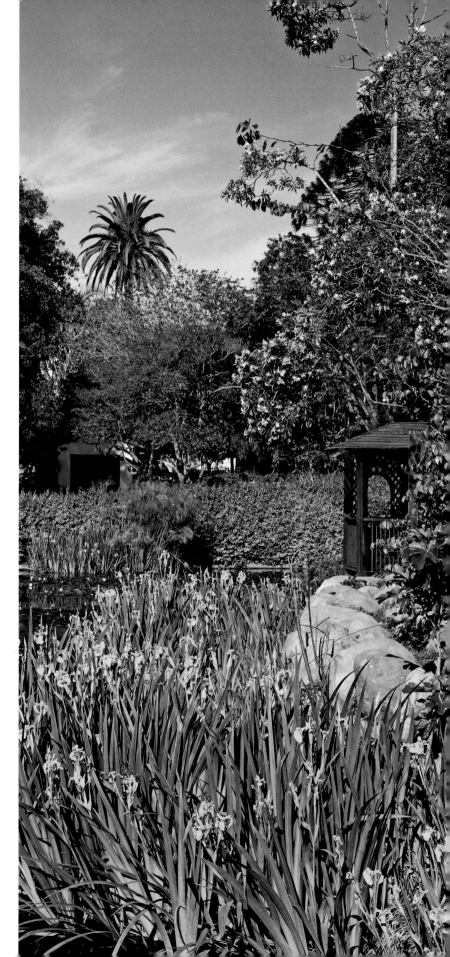

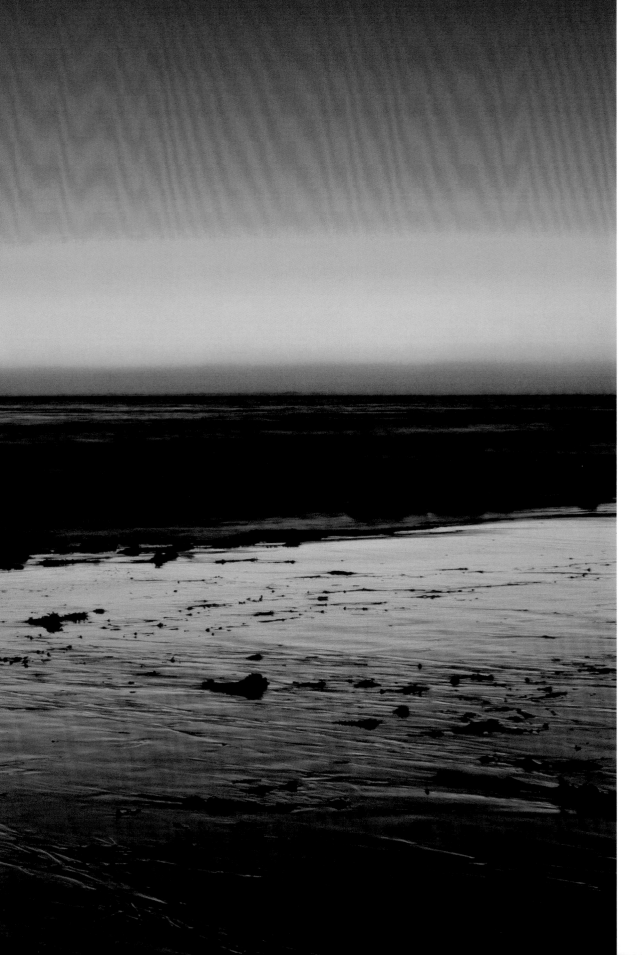

Caring for the body is like tending to the garden. We must pull the weeds, water the plants, and rake the beds. Tremendous patience is required. We hardly work alone, though, and our efforts resume each morning as the sun warms the evening's damp cover. To sit in the shade, to touch the dirt, to trim and weed—I helped this garden grow.

In my own experience with chronic pain and elusive symptoms, it was difficult to find a doctor who would listen, and even more difficult to find one who would teach me how to heal. I realize I had always pushed my physical self toward a "performance model" without accepting my body as a system. One part of healing is the patient's understanding of her condition, but the relationship between individual and cosmos that I found along the seashore and in the garden gave me the acceptance I needed to take care of myself.

—Dana

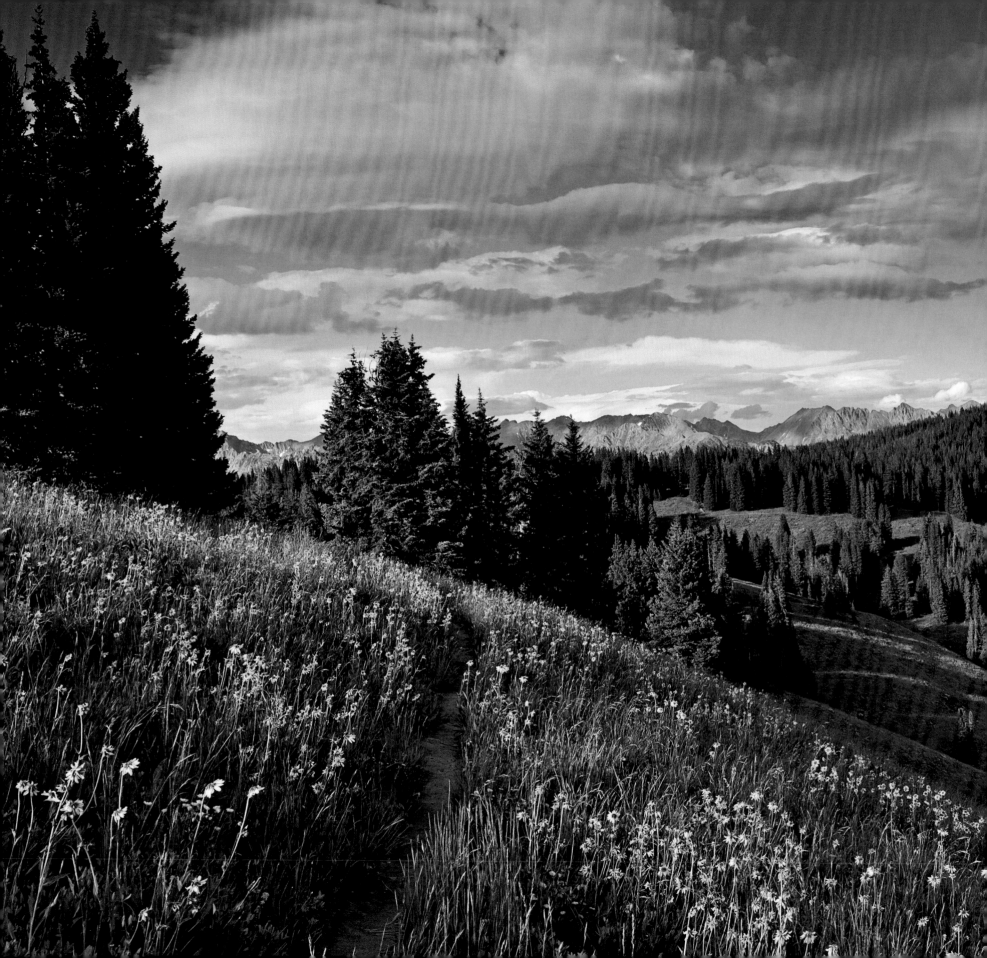

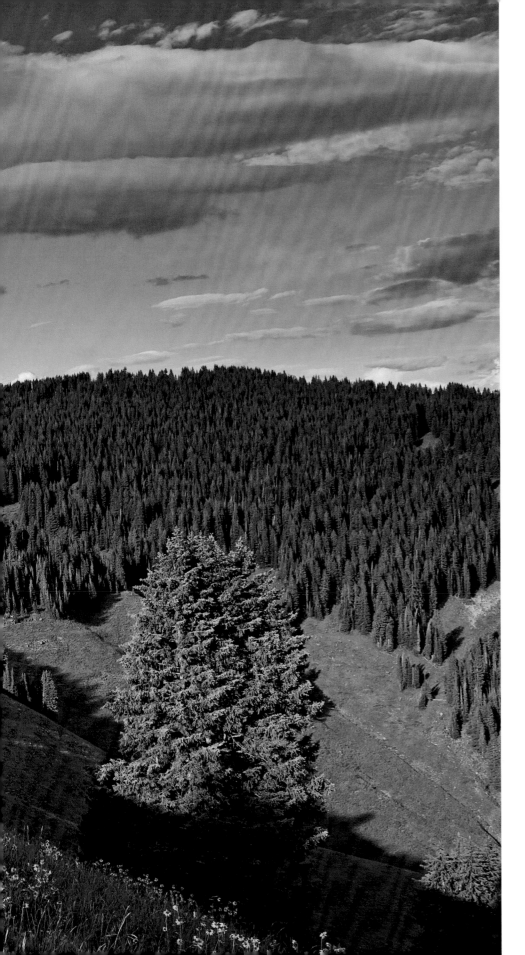

Reaching Out
Vail, Colorado

I can't believe I'm here, that I've put myself with all these others with multiple sclerosis for a week in Vail, Colorado. Jimmy Heuga himself, ski champion of the '60s, had founded this center after his diagnosis ten years earlier, 1975. Contrary to modern- and limited-medical belief that bed rest was the preferable management technique, Heuga had pushed himself to discover his personal limits, the same as he had done in his professional racing. Jimmy and his team taught us to take charge, that we could and should move.

So soon after my diagnosis, even though my arm and hand still weren't quite "right," didn't perform basic tasks like open door when asked or sign my name, I certainly wasn't disabled like all the others. I walked into the room unassisted, no cane or walker.

I also came alone, no caretaker or spouse. Why did I think I could do this alone? Because I craved information and believed the Vail mountains would care for me. They'd been my favored slopes for many seasons of skiing. Now as I sat among these other multiple sclerosis patients, I wasn't sure at all, not sure I could look at my own possible or probable future of immobility. I read the statistics: Only one in three is wheelchair bound by the end. Over half move on from relapsing-remitting multiple sclerosis to progressive. But these numbers aren't encouraging. I had signed in hoping to gain personal advice on nutrition and exercise along with guidelines for relationships and work. Easing my discomfort of fearful possibilities, Jimmy Heuga himself was among us, and he'd recently married despite his increasing disabilities. No one told me I'd get better, that I wouldn't end up in a wheelchair, but they were all saying get up and do, whatever you can. Being in a wheelchair isn't a death sentence; and, as I saw the joyful expressions on other faces, who were encountering hope for the first time or reuniting with old friends from previous sessions, I knew I couldn't quit.

These others with multiple sclerosis were in different stages, but they had all come to this clinic to hope for more, more acceptance and maybe more ability. Some came just to be among others who were disabled … for these days no one is looking askance at jerky arms, unwieldy legs that have to be assisted as foreign objects onto wheelchair frames. I don't worry that my hand looks more like a claw than human hand. This older gal next to me has trouble speaking, can't mouth the words correctly, but she's happy to be here. That I know from her companion. It's her third year here. Will I also continue to return, year by year growing in disability, and somehow still able to be grateful?

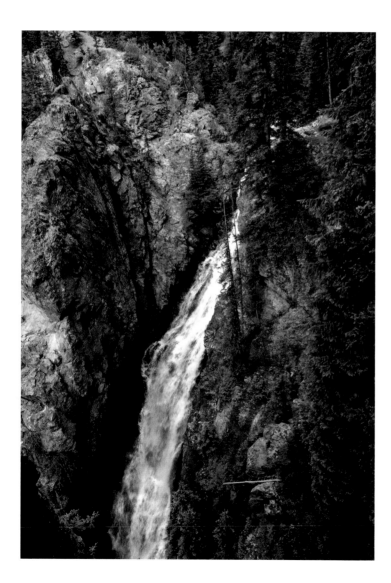

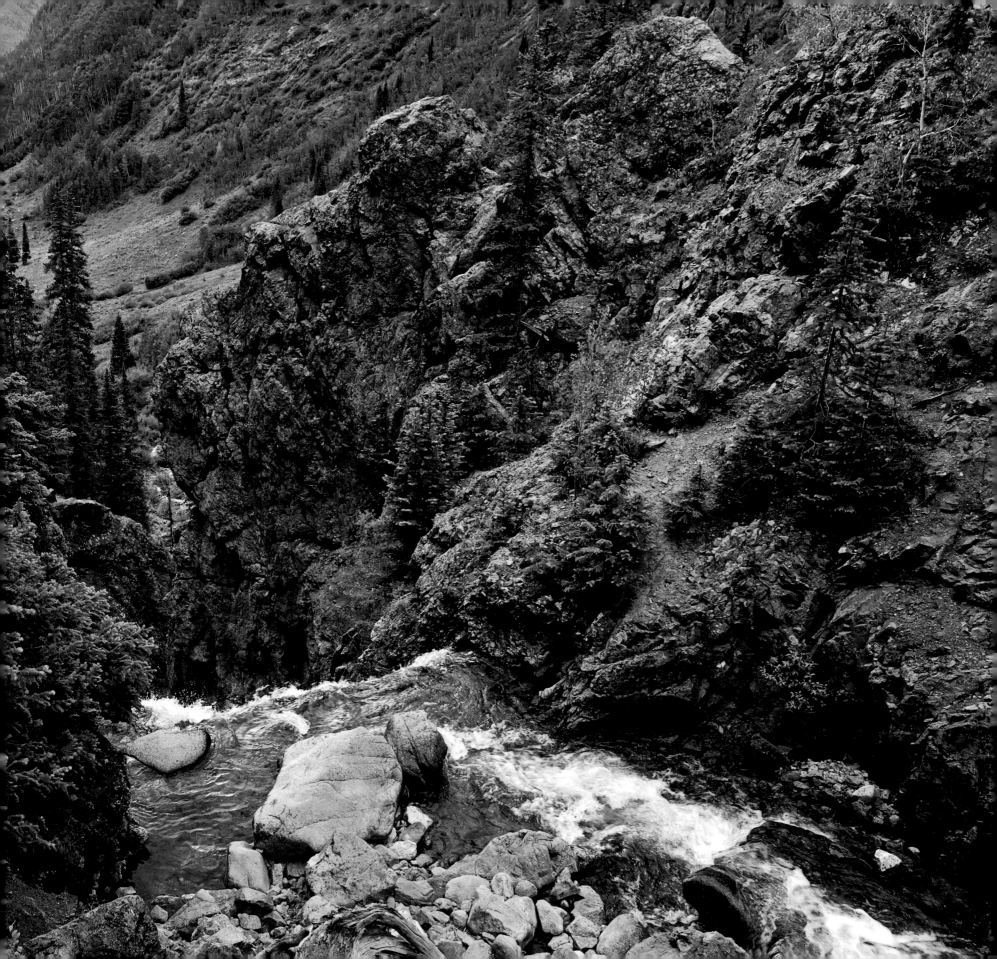

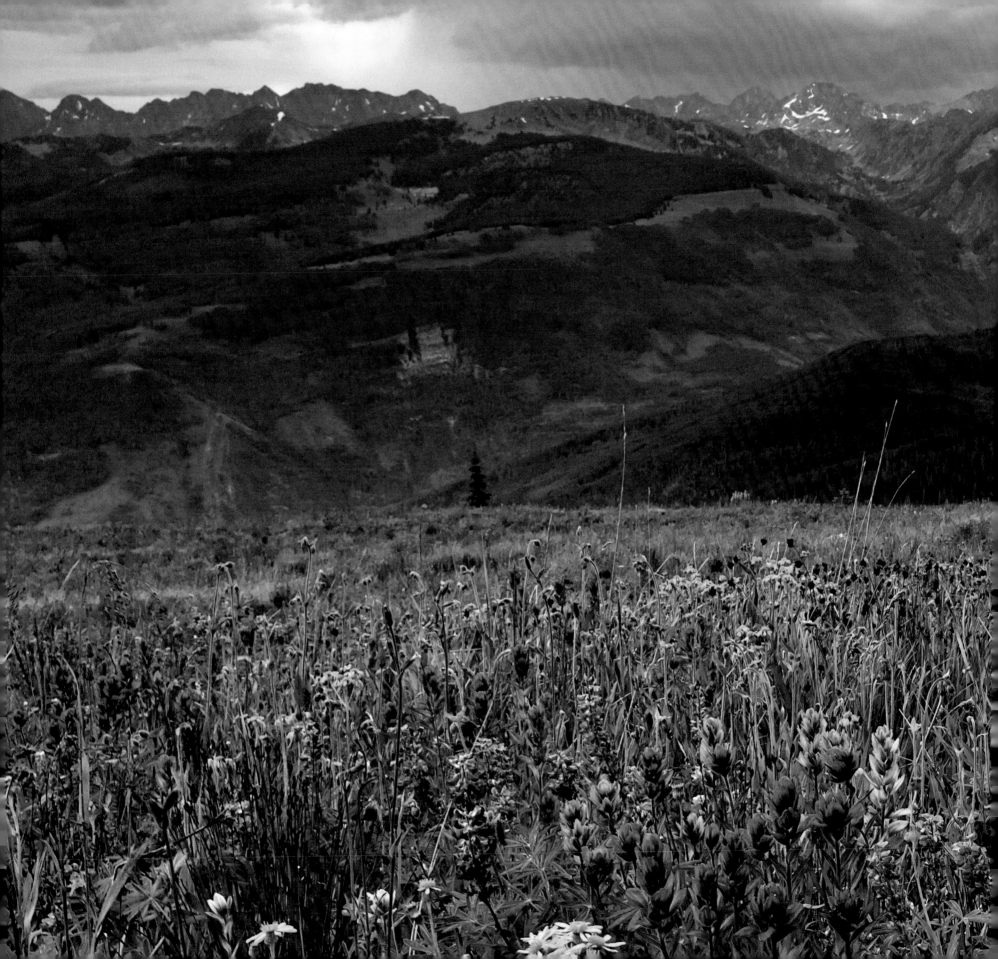

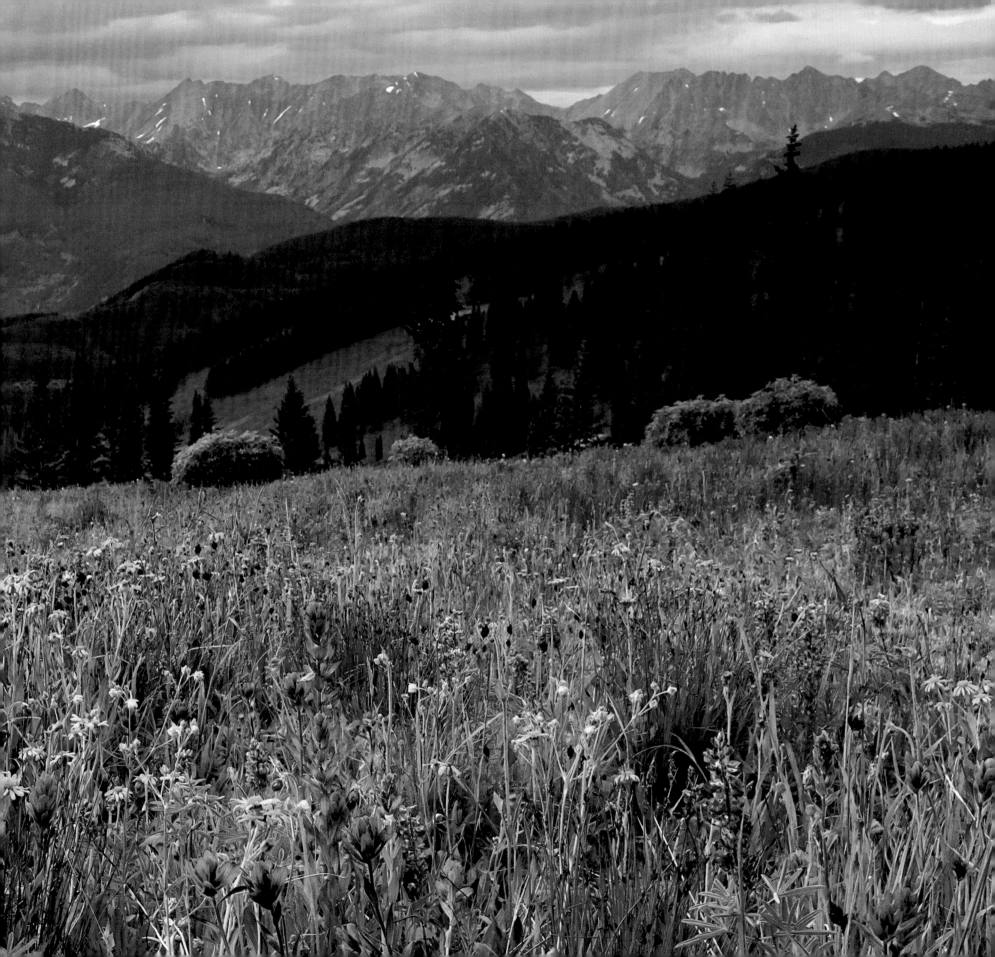

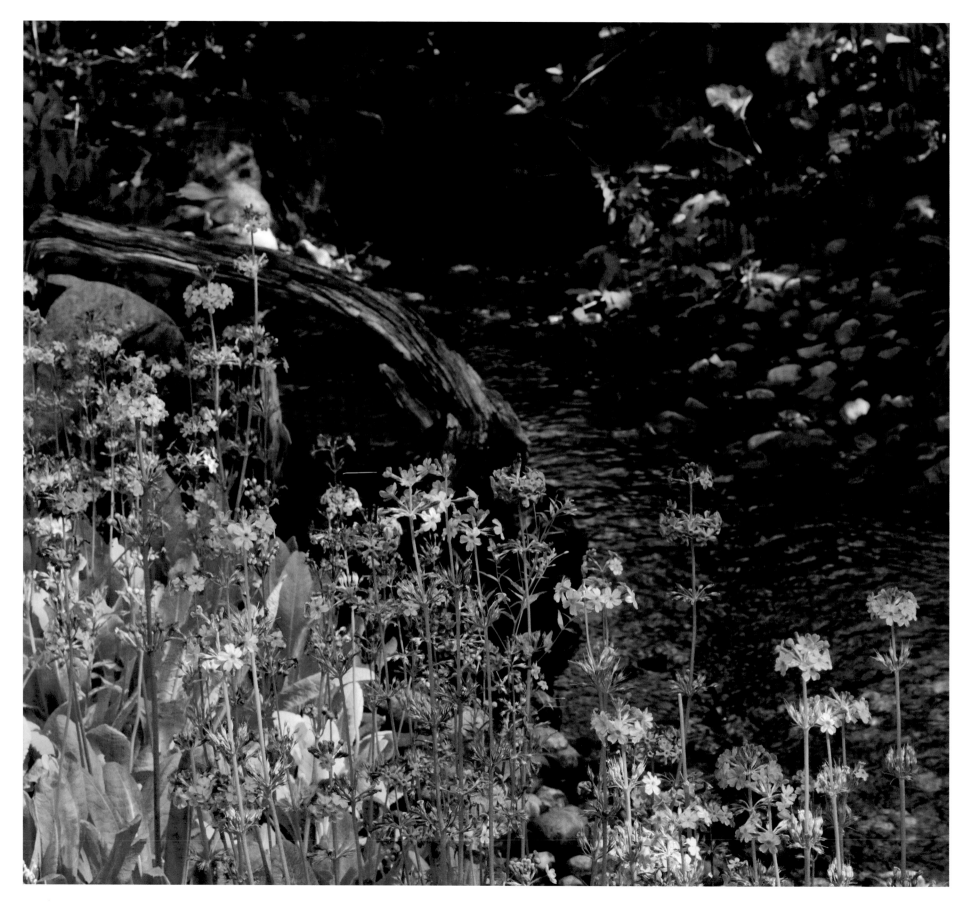

Jimmy doesn't promise a thing, but his example speaks volumes. Even in advanced stages of this disease inspiration is possible. My success as director of research in a money management firm in New York City was no preparation for this, but maybe my earlier years had prepared me. Maybe just living in New York City had given me the same fortitude to carry on that Jimmy had gained in his years training for ski racing. For both of us our minds and spirits were stronger than our bodies, our inner resources enough.

But my feelings still threatened me that I was alone. Yet I wanted to be alone. It was my choice to deal with my body and my condition on my own. No one else could understand what it was like, but at the clinic they could. I continued comparing myself to them—that I was younger, 39; that I could walk unaided; I could feed myself. I never denied that I shared the same disease. Being there alone gave me the chance to discover my own way of living with multiple sclerosis. I had memories of these mountains, of gliding down their slopes in perfect snow. I felt I belonged there after decades of skiing.

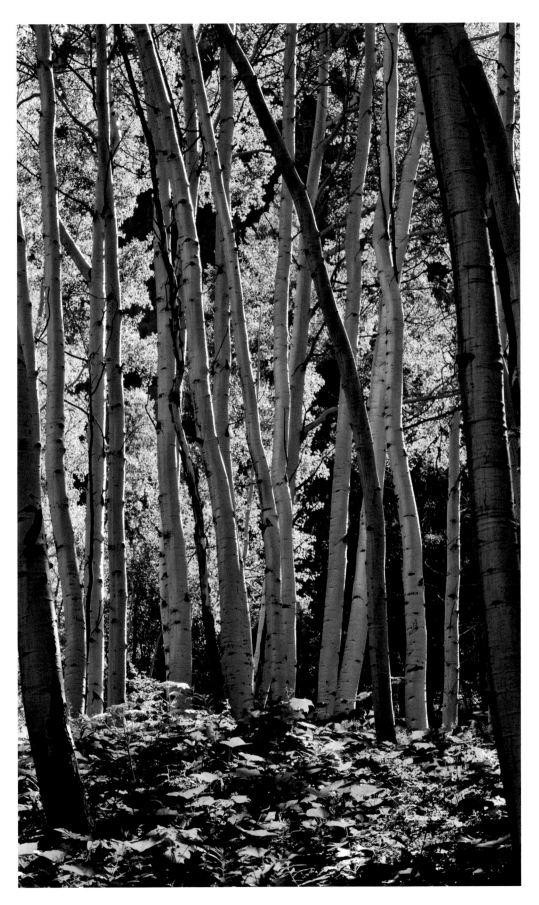

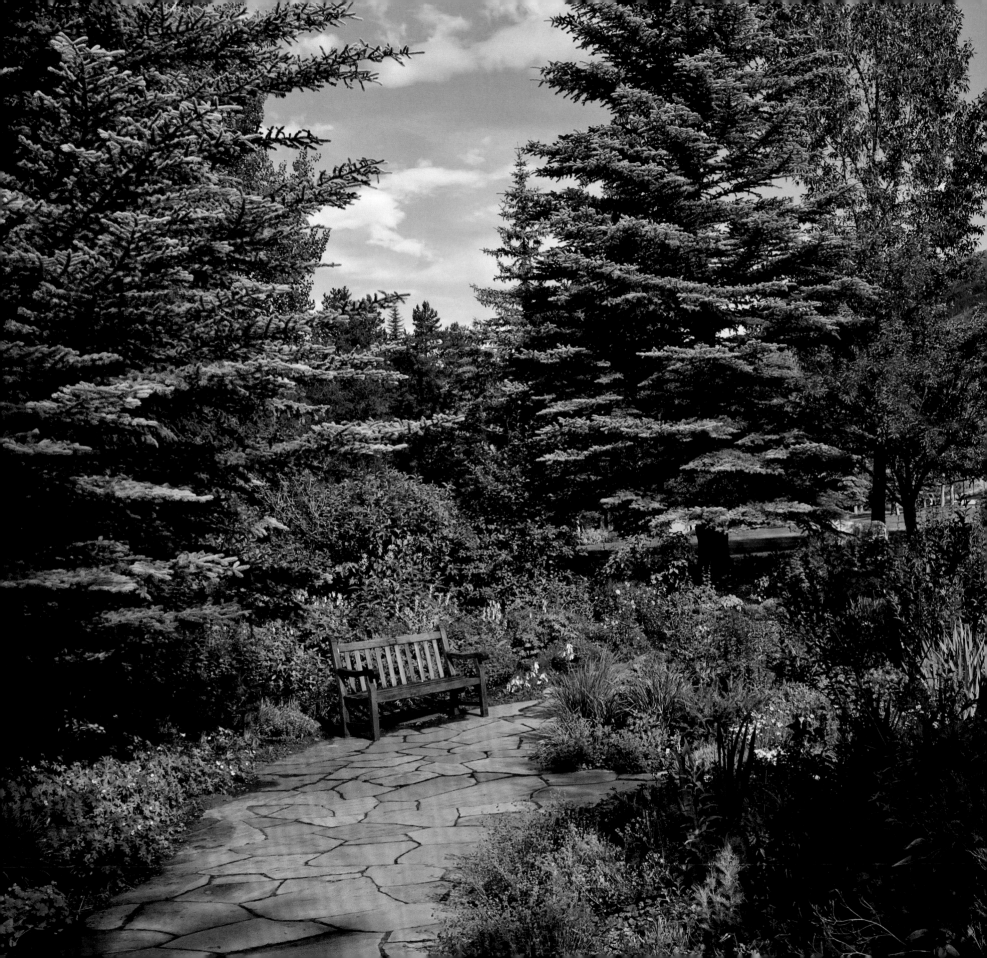

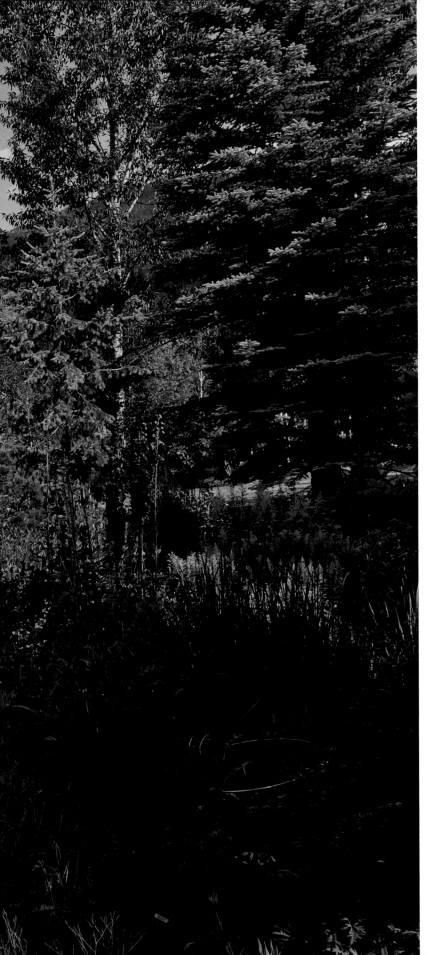

I slipped away from the lecture hall after dinner, wanting the solace of the peaks and brisk air. The trees, fragrant in the early summer, were different from the snow-laden branches of wintertime. I had never really noticed them before; skiing they were obstacles to avoid. Now they still stood tall, barely moving. Their naked presence was reassuring, their just being. I knew then that I would continue in this fight to have a full life; maybe without skis, but I could and would continue. Somehow there would always be an outside in nature for comfort.

As I rejoined the others, I listened with a new attentiveness. The messages were for me. Yes my body in exercise needed to stay cool to keep my core temperature down or symptoms might reappear; my balance might always be tricky. I was glad to leave the Jimmy Heuga Clinic with a lot of new information, neurologic and physiologic, helpful advice on relationships and honestly sharing. But more important to me, I came away with a new awareness of Nature abiding. A deep wisdom had touched me outside that night.

—Karen

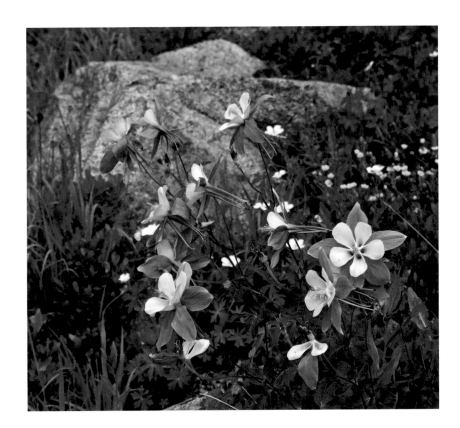

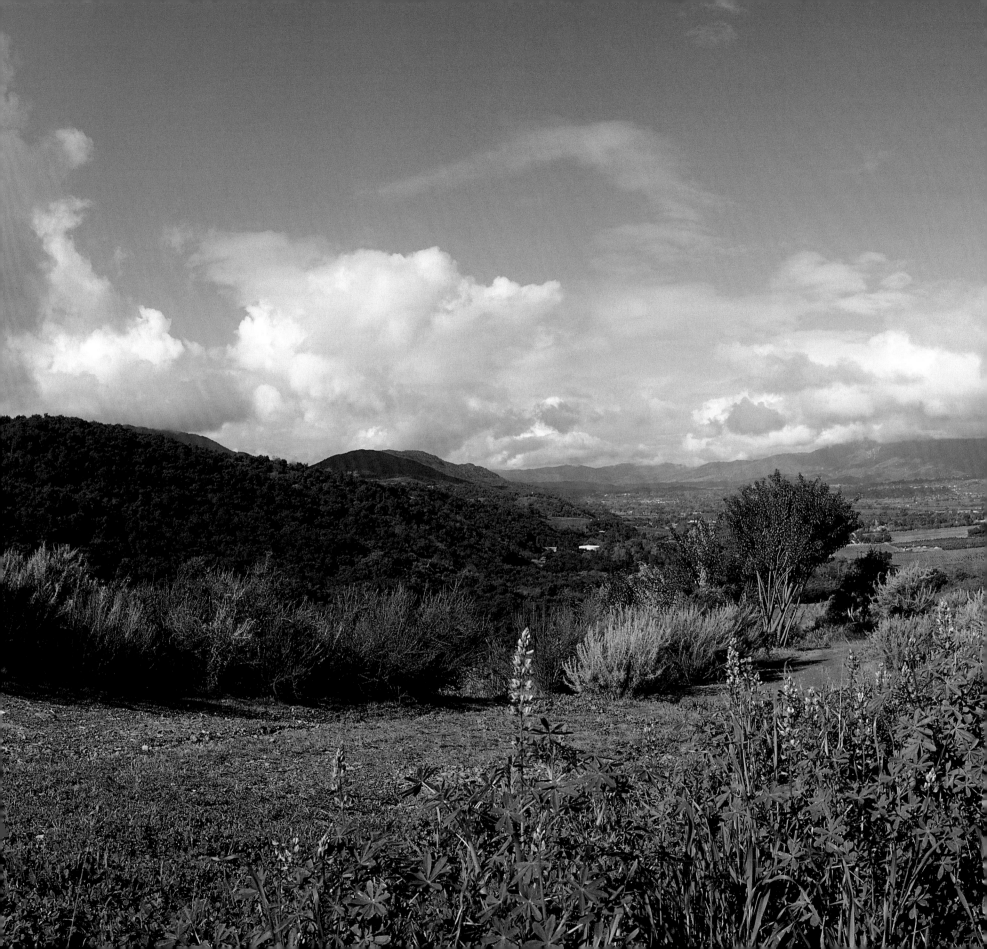

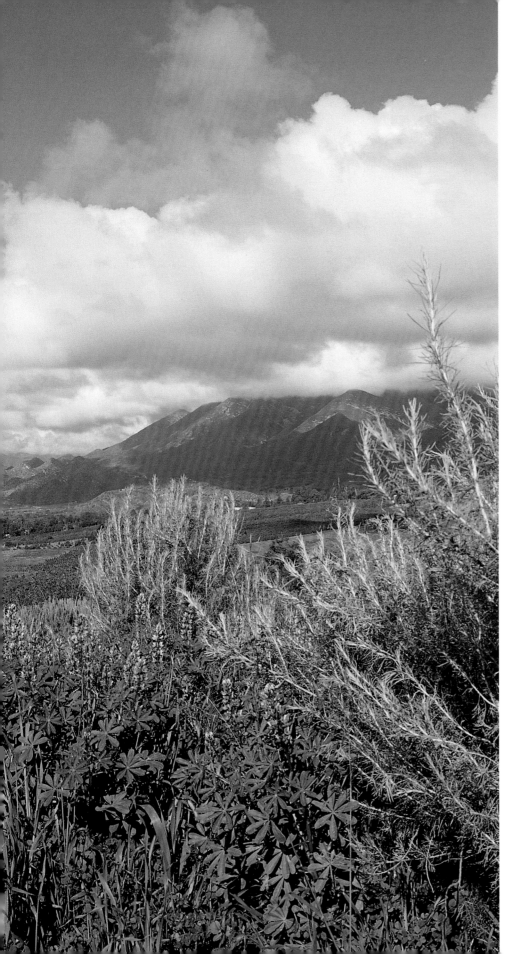

Diagnosis to Freedom
Ojai, California

I was referred to a doctor in Ojai, after so many had given up. He ordered the tests that diagnosed the Lyme disease. Finally, I had an explanation. It was with tremendous relief that I could now identify a condition and connect it to the symptoms I had suffered. The New York doctor who told me at the onset of my ailments to try and relax could finally be cast off. I was no longer required to bear the burden of his frustrating advice to "just take some yoga classes." My mind began to wrap itself around a decade of fatigue, night sweats, irritable bowel syndrome, body aches, and depression.

With new information in hand, I turned to the Internet to find stories of recovery. I quickly connected with others who had already found answers. I realized my body had been compromised by this infection; internal systems, from adrenal to immune, were exhausted and would take time to replenish.

What I remember most from my visits to the Ojai medical clinic was the drive from Santa Barbara. After turning off the hectic and crowded 101 Freeway, I began a gentle glide along Casitas Pass. Each time, I would slip into this valley and turn on a CD of Native American flute music. As my body relaxed, the warmth of the music carried my spirit into a protected, womb-like space.

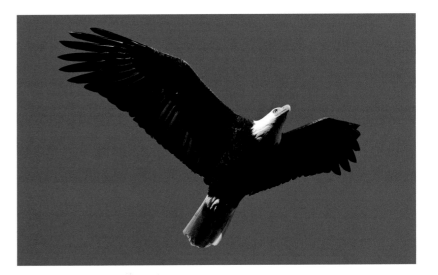

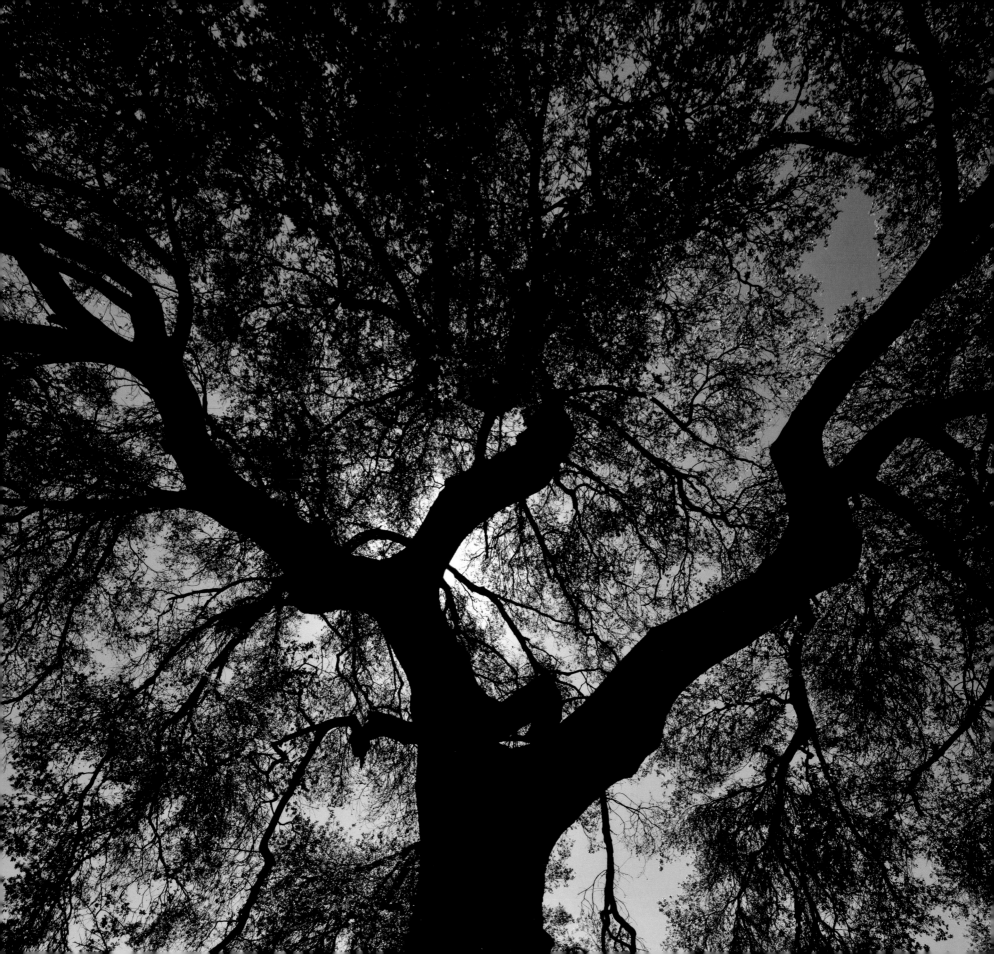

Solitary oaks on the rolling hills spoke to me. I gazed at the places where they grew, appreciating the beauty. I marveled at their independence and strength. Branches opened massive canopies of leaf, providing shade on the sunny slopes. The trees seemed to shy from hilltops and preferred the terrain tucked between. I have read that oaks were often the center for meetings and worship and were sacred to many gods: the Norse Thor, the Roman Jupiter, the Slavic Perun, the Celtic Dagda, and the Hebrew El.

After years of feeling fragile and adrift, I yearned to feel rooted and strong like the oaks. I began to include a bodywork session after each medical treatment. At first, it was extremely difficult to have someone touch my body. Living so long without a diagnosis had made me feel toxic, as if I might bring harm or pain to those I encountered. The hands of a massage therapist allowed a sensory connection that had been broken. It took many visits to get back "into my skin." I realized the importance of feeling the tender, painful parts. During one session, I accepted that pain was in my body, and at the same time my perspective shifted. I realized my body is so much larger than the pain. This helped me experience the space that surrounded this tightness so that I could let it go.

There is a flower stand along Casitas Pass. Payment is deposited in a tin box. I never stopped, but I would daydream as I drove by. I imagined a woman selecting fresh flowers from the field below, arranging simple bouquets, and leaving them to be collected by visitors. Perhaps, the first rays of daylight reached her face as she returned to the morning chores. This became a landmark in a way, dependable and steadfast. I needed to find a few constants, as I opened to changes within. Meditation and swimming were providing a deepening connection between body and mind. For now, this flower stand represented something pure and helped me believe in the possibility of my own return to health.

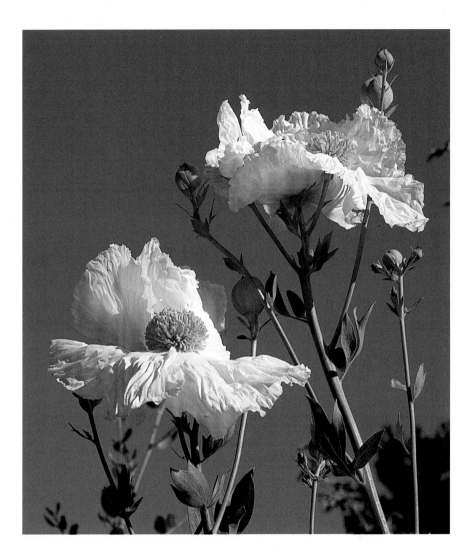

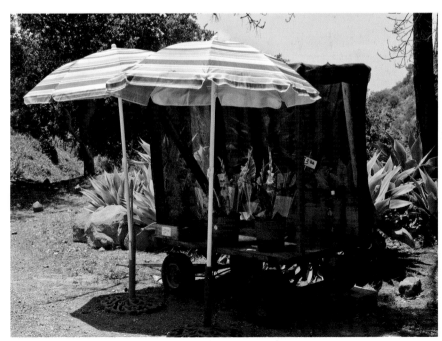

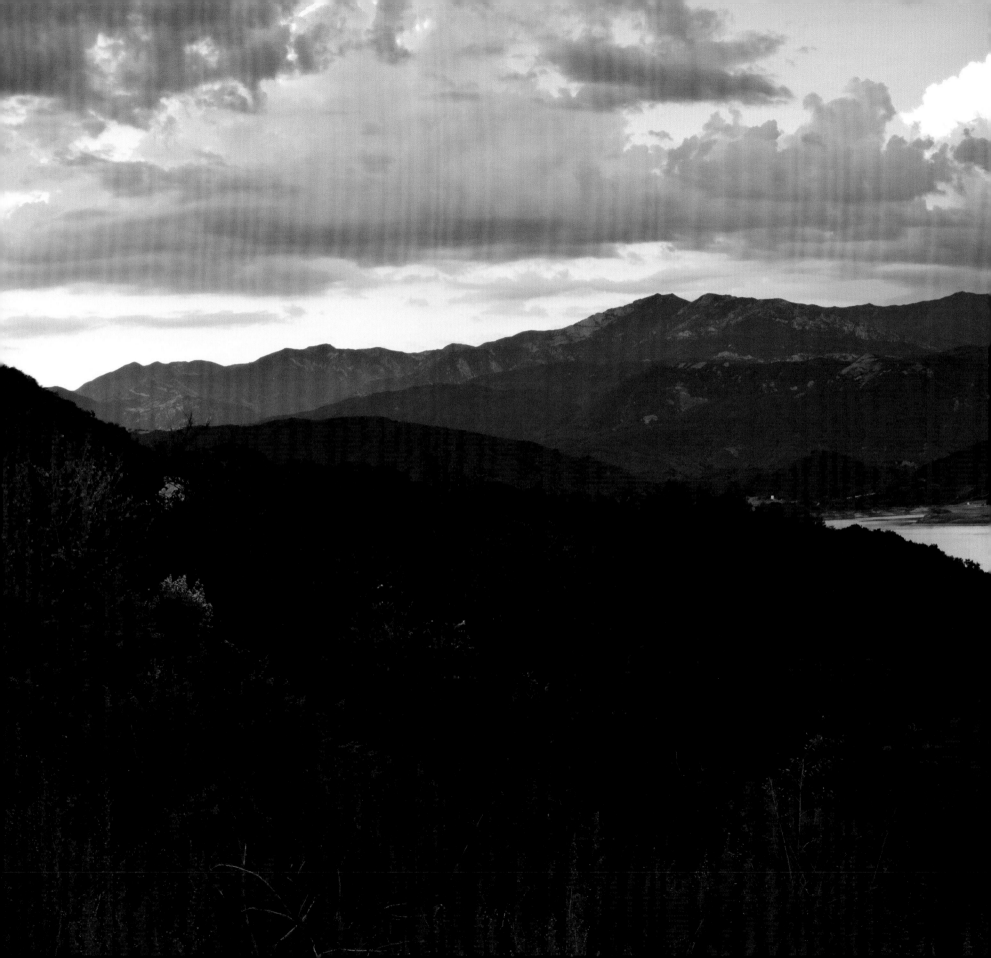

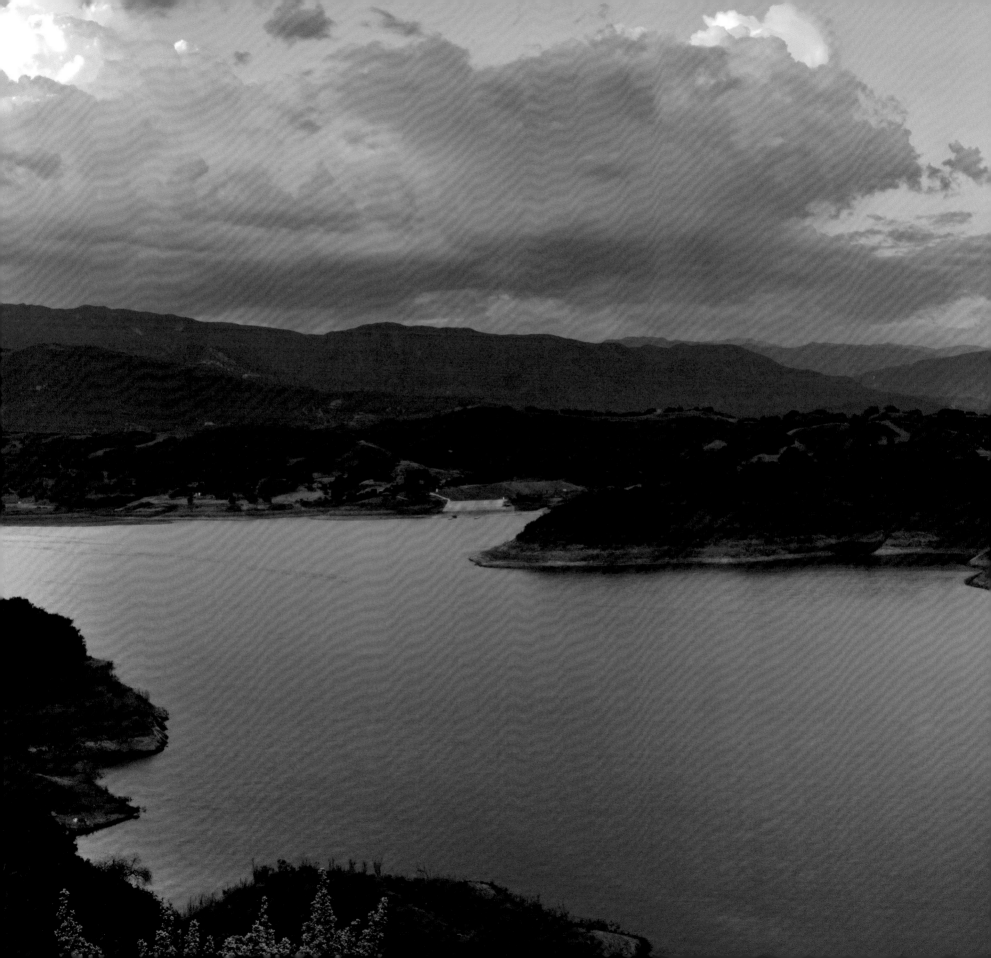

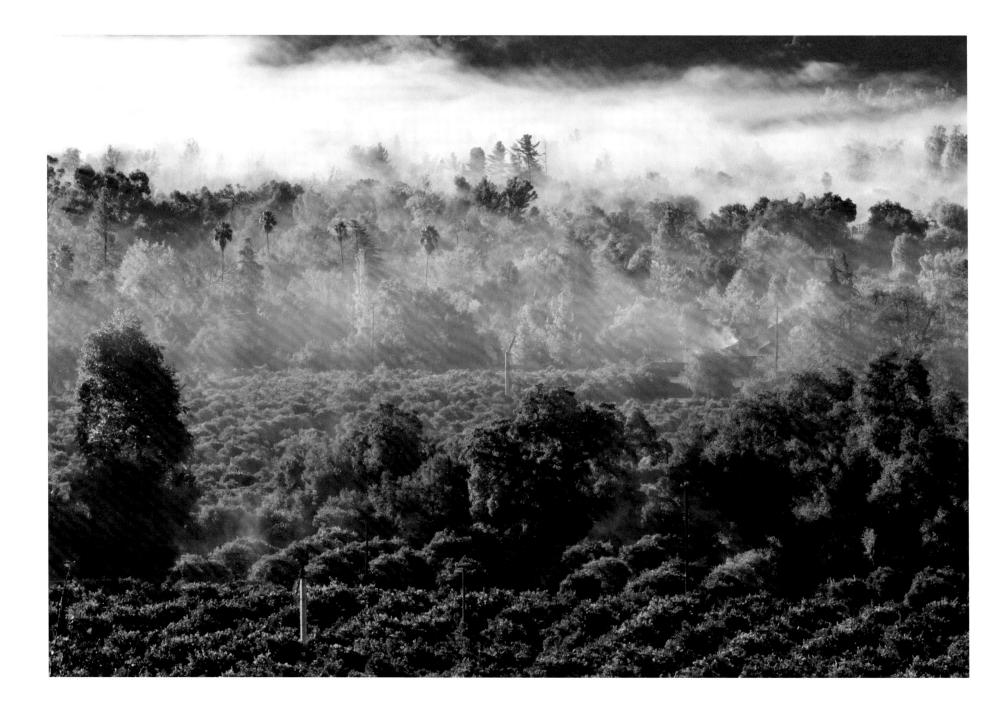

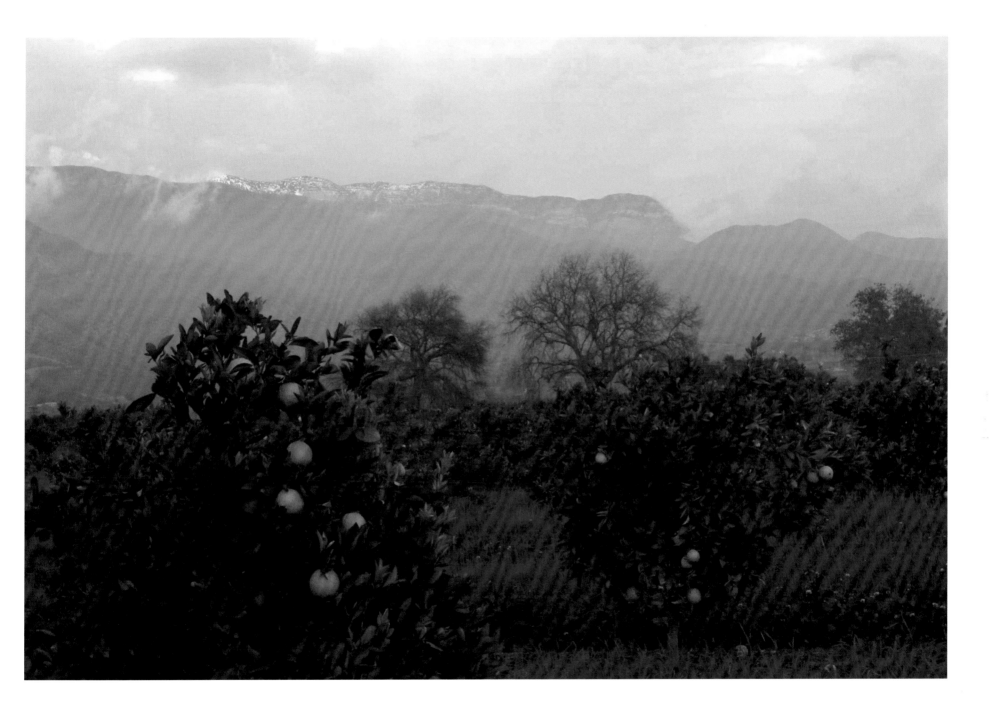

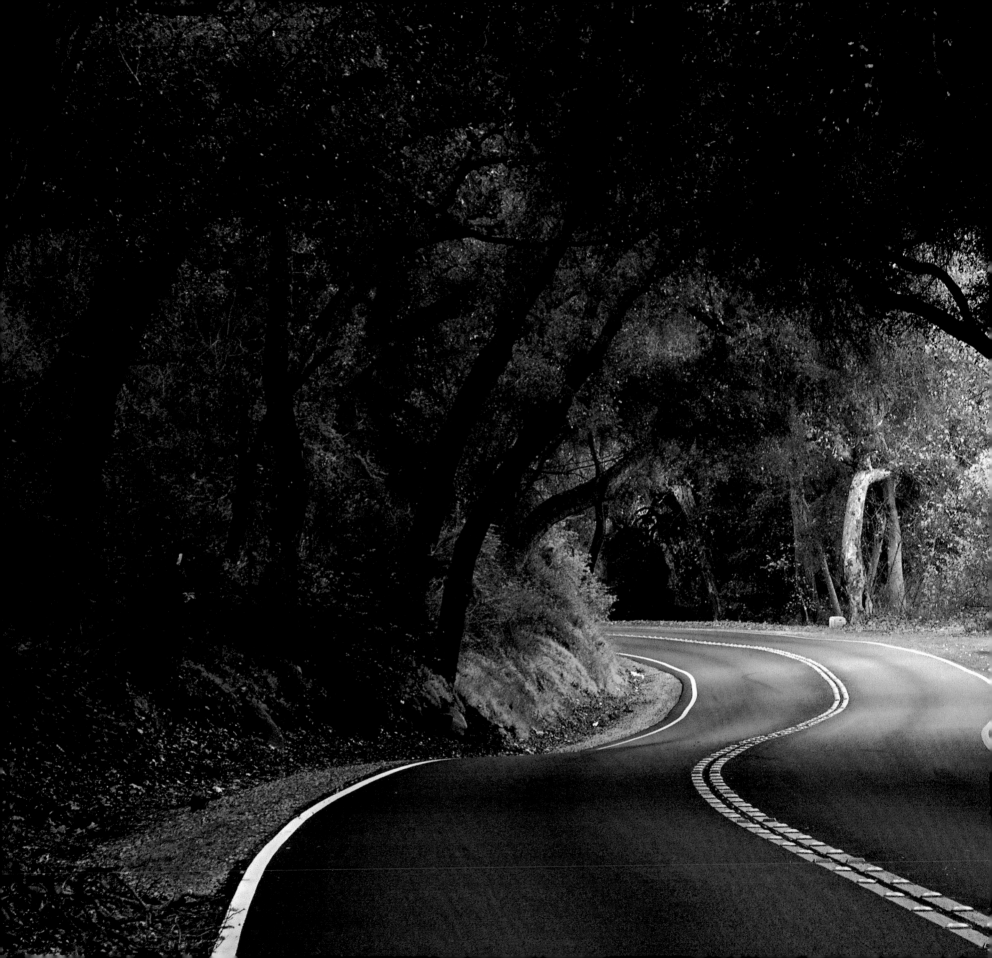

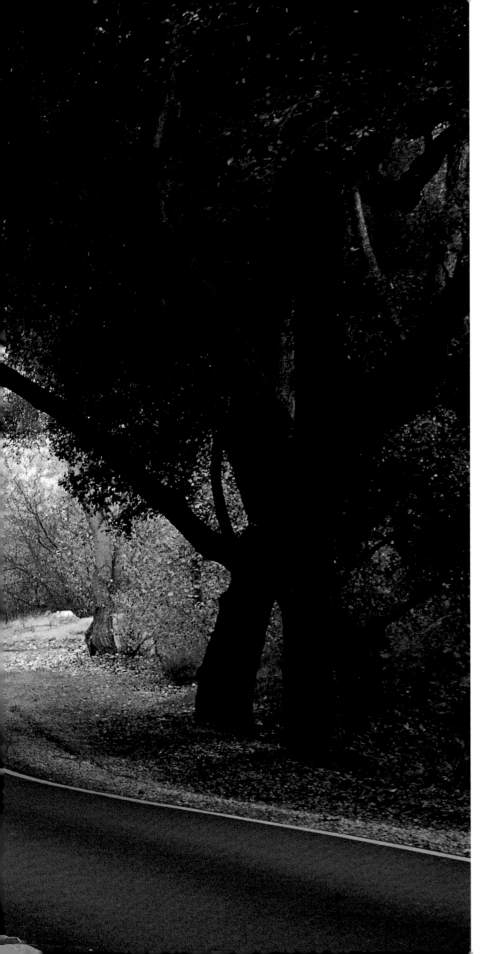

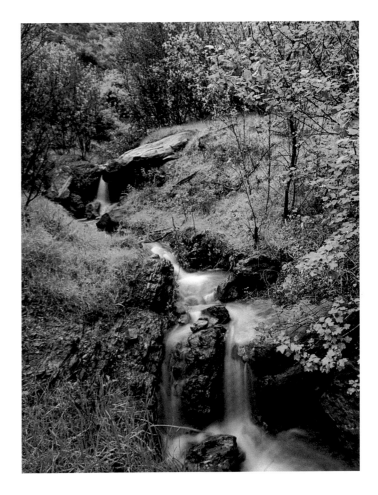

As I improved, I found opportunities to volunteer. Sometimes these offerings were rather simple: a phone call to a neighbor or a short letter to a friend. Eventually I would devote my time to a soup kitchen, youth program, and public garden. These acts of service allowed me to regain a sense of purpose and value. I came to understand health on levels beyond the physical. My journey along Casitas Pass had encouraged me to imagine my next destination in life.

—Dana

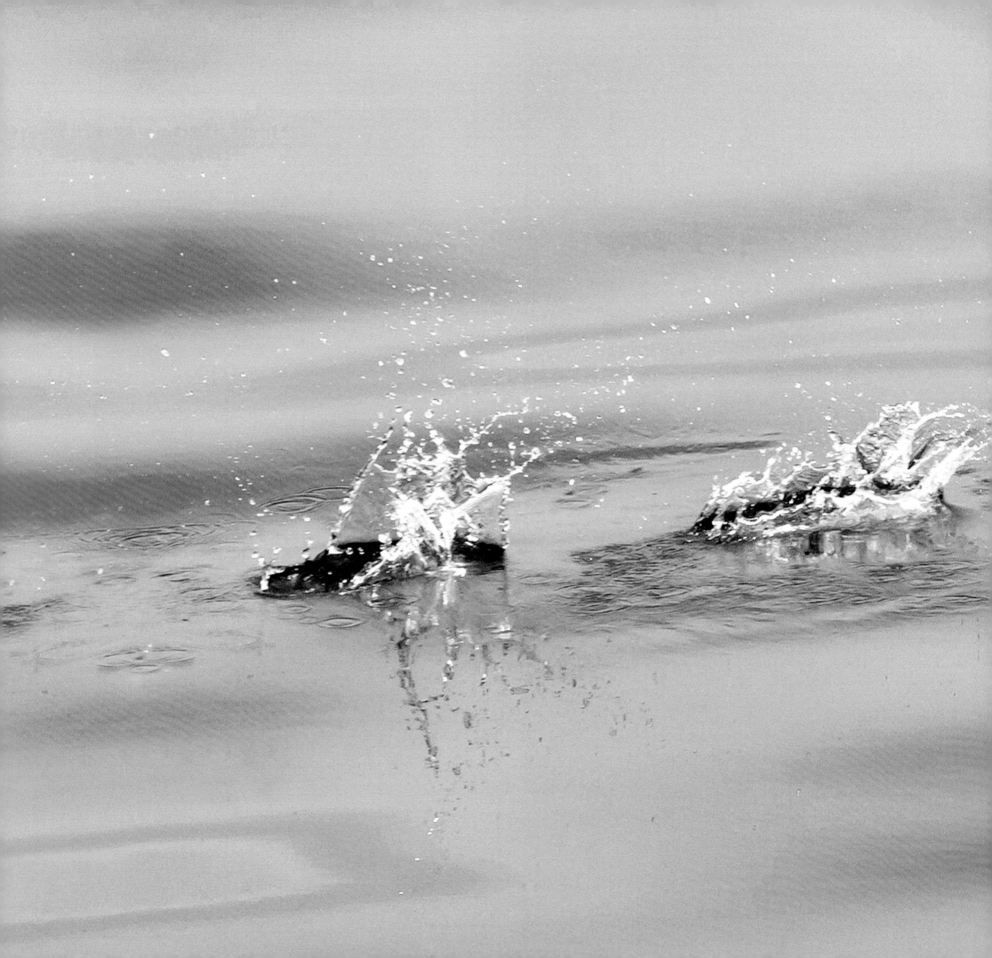

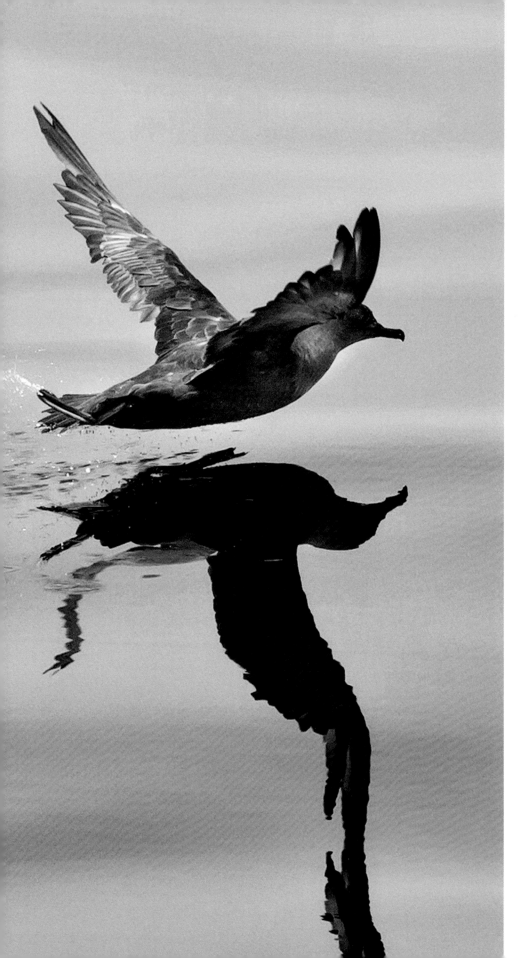

Surfacing
Goleta, California

When my leg injury ended my daily bicycle ride, I was told to go to the water. Swimming had never been a strong sport for me: I never liked getting my hair wet, never found speed in my stroke. Thus, I reluctantly jumped into the pool. The water received me. Entering the pool in the dark became a morning ritual. The sky would gradually lighten, as clouds were emblazoned with shades of pink and orange. I would alternate between freestyle and backstroke, watching colors brighten. One of the many aspects I appreciated about swimming was the fact that no swim was ever the same. My body, mood, the water were always changing.

The aqueous environment provided a space to reintegrate movement without the hindrance of pain. Each lap was a goal reached. I could also float and be carried by a marvelous, weightless sensation. The water was strong and yielding, calming and supportive. I connected with the swing of arm and leg—each dependent on the other appendage to gracefully glide out of the way. I realized I needed to allow flexibility to flow into all aspects of my life. Some mornings the pool was very busy with many kicking, horizontal bodies. Despite the crowd, I found my own speed, and acceleration increased. I wondered if the additional bodies and waves they generated were affecting the buoyancy. It was as if we were each contributing to the power of the other.

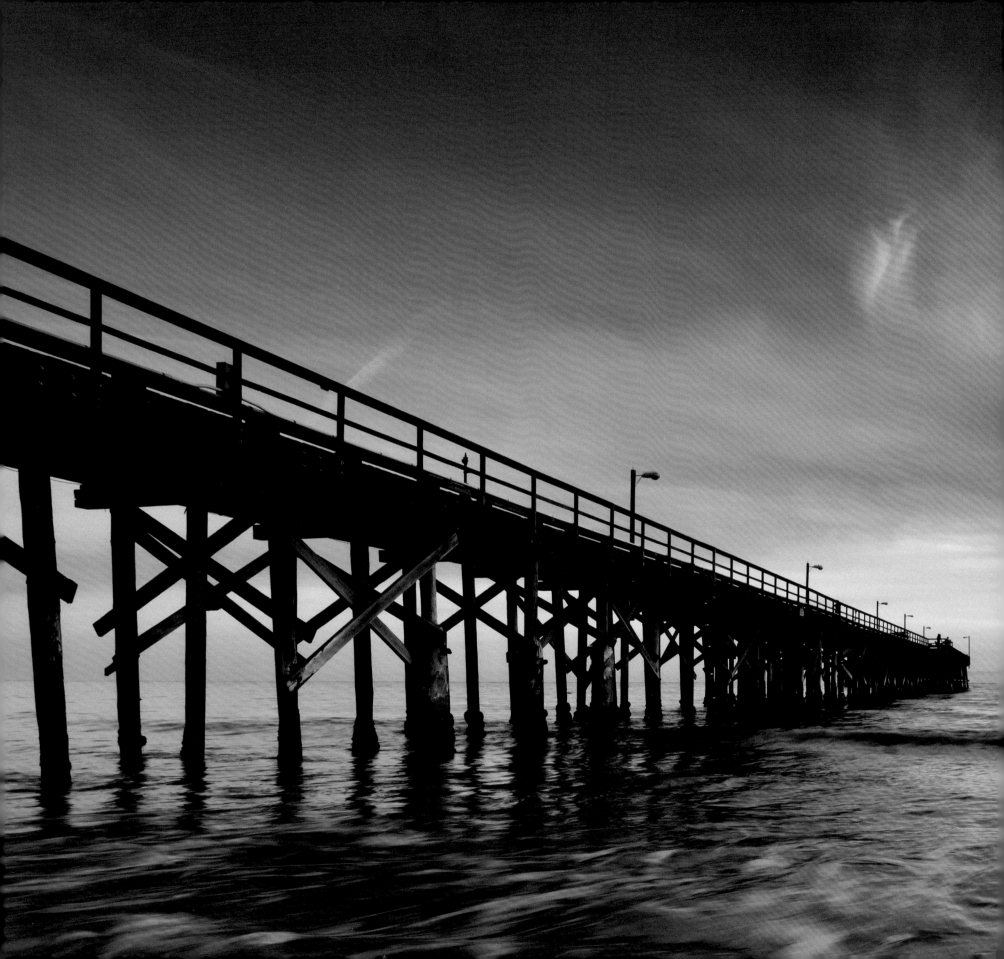

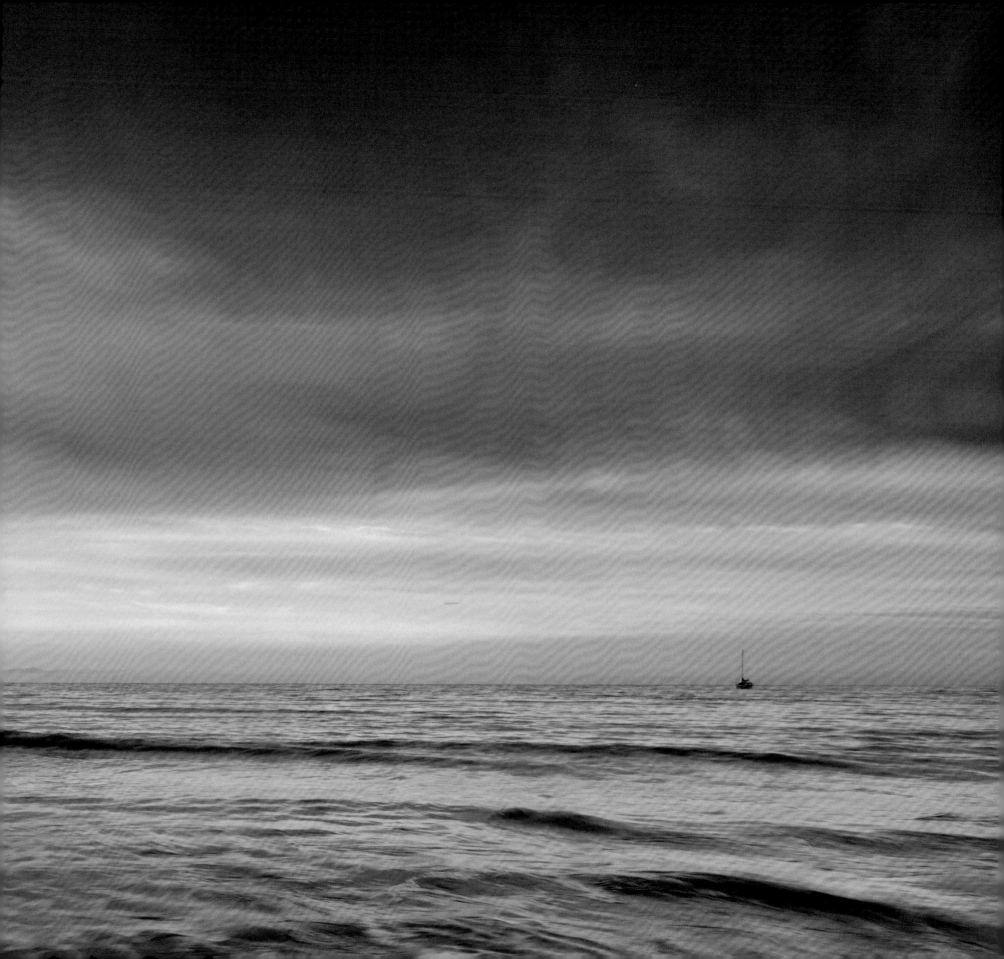

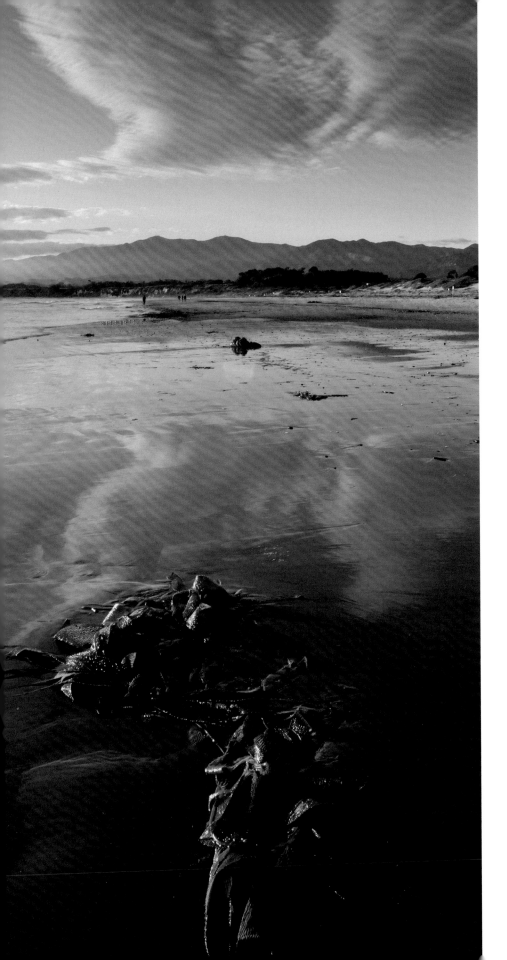

While swimming in the rain, there is this terrific moment of uncertainty when you lift your head, almost a vertigo effect, and you are gripped by one question: Am I below or above the surface? There is no distinction, just water. Underneath the rippling surface, the water below feels quiet and protected. Emerging again, you discover a melody of water playing water. I loved swimming in the rain. As the falling raindrops merged with the water that surrounded me, I remembered once reading that every molecule of every droplet of water in existence today has always been there. Every droplet in this pool had a story to tell!

As I moved my head, turning below, then turning above, I considered how my body was integrating water and air through my exercise. This feeling of active unity, centered on my physical being, pushed me to consider how I might align my career and professional search with my unique gifts and interests. Swimming continually taught me to expand and to consider new options. Like the two red-tailed hawks I so often watched, circles join; they separate; they are parallel; then they fuse; they expand and contract; there are two; there is one. My mind and imagination were opening.

On one occasion, a spectacular winged creature caught my eye. I could not tell if it was a hummingbird or giant moth. It circled in play and then landed directly in front of me on the lane buoy. There we were—two creatures floating in the water. Face-to-face, I admired my visitor's brown-and-peach wings. The animal had crawled inside the plastic buoy, and I was quickly realizing this was not an aquatic creature. I reached out my finger, and it climbed aboard, gripping my finger with legs that seemed to have little thorn-like toes running up and down them. Together, we got out of the pool, and I placed the creature on a plant. Had I done the right thing? I could not identify the animal, nor did I know where it belonged. It seemed happy in air, on land, and in water. Perhaps, it had come to the water with a purpose I did not realize. Had I done harm? In the shower, I cried.

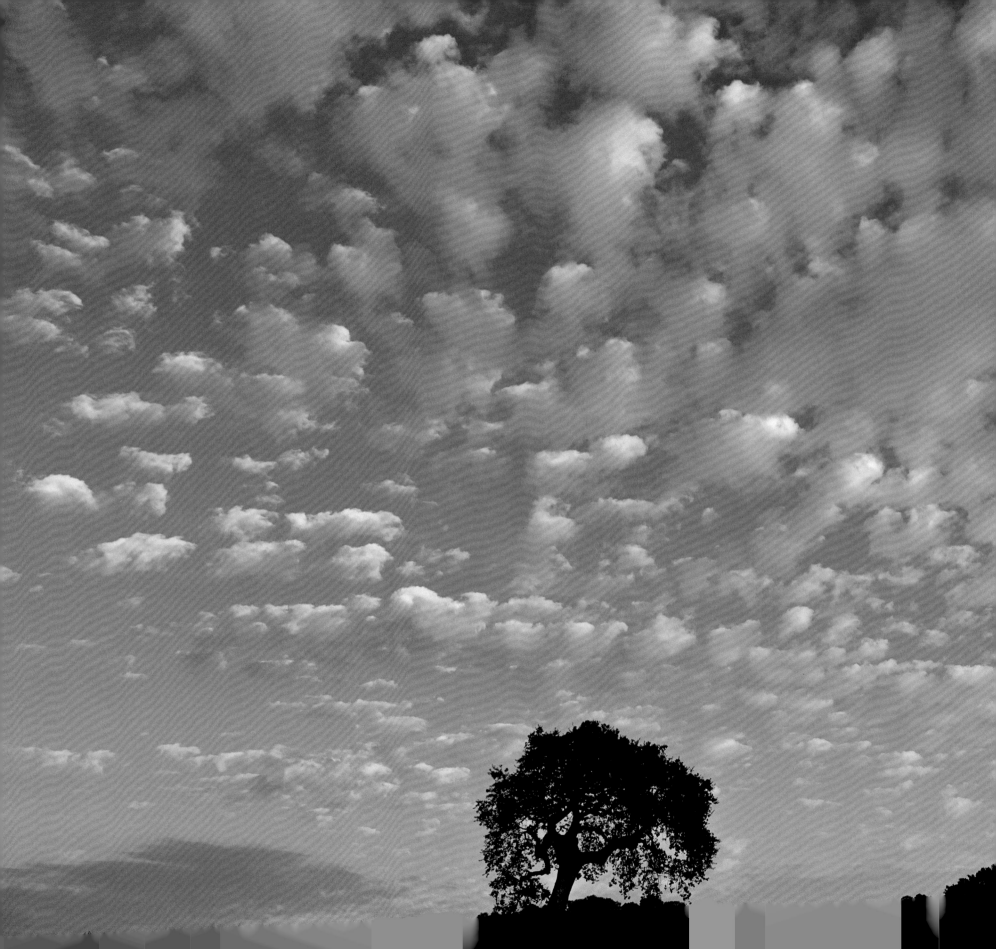

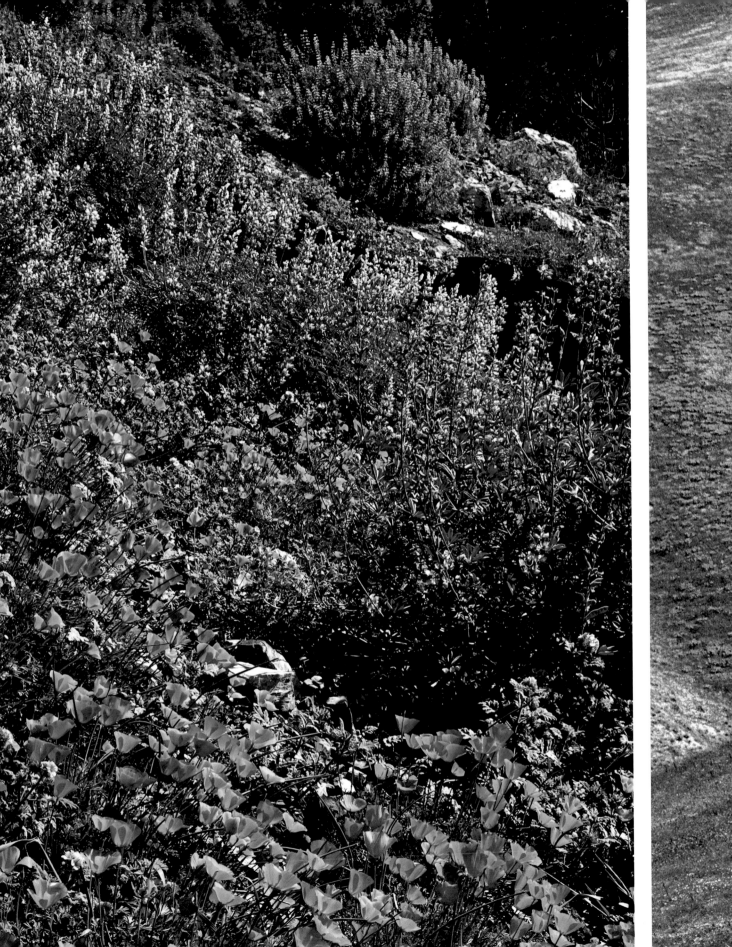
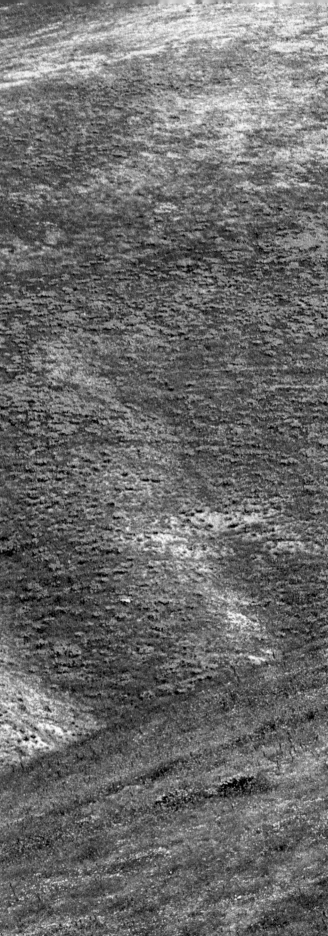

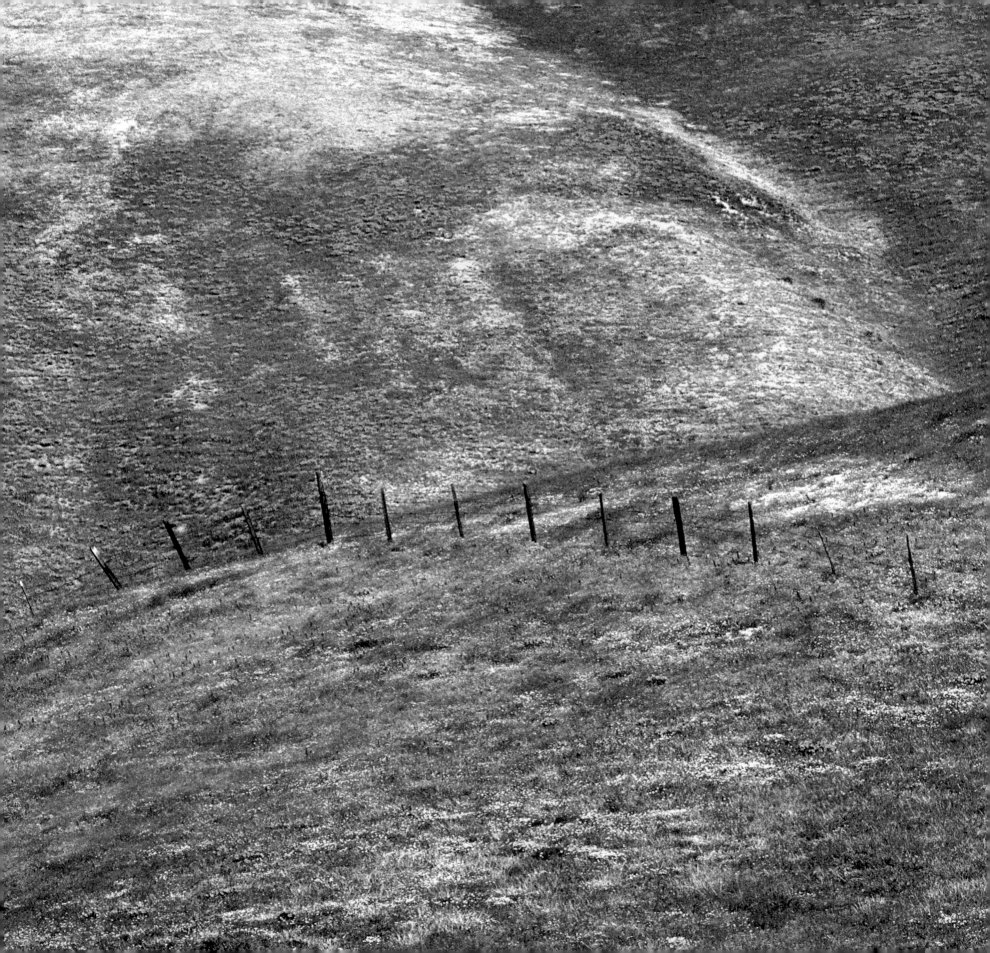

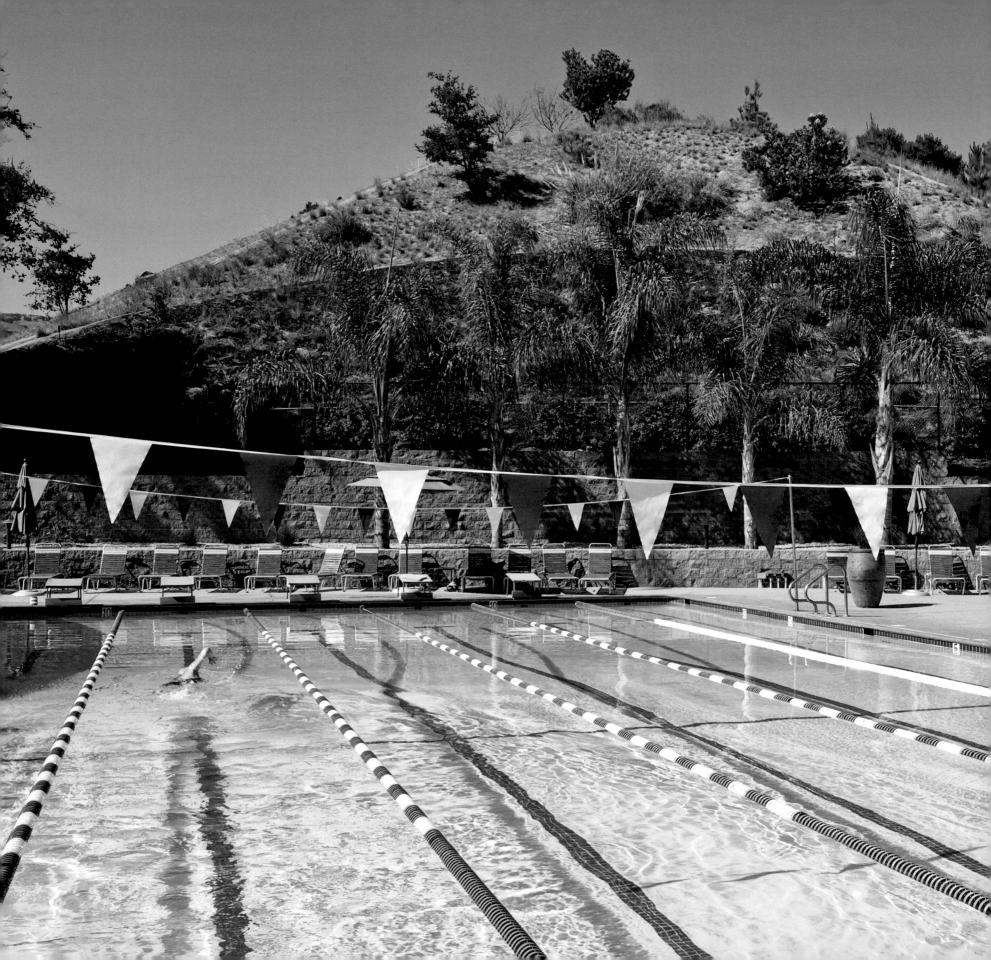

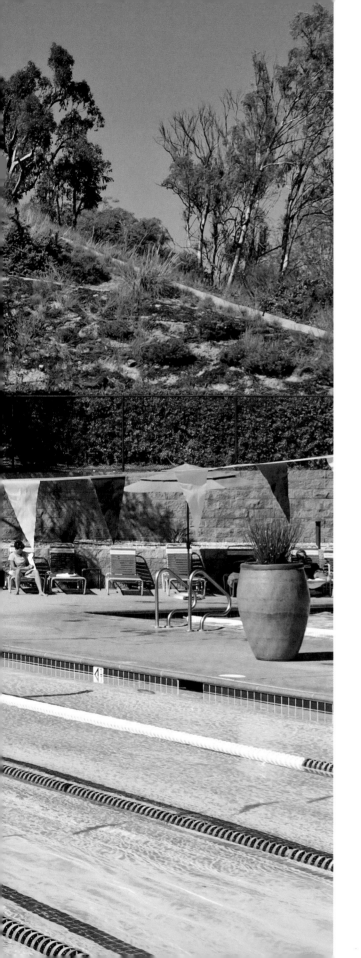

My sickness had caused a rather paralyzing fear that I would disappoint people or be unable to fulfill an obligation or promise. I had come to doubt my own ability to take care of myself and thus questioned all my actions. When sickness befalls us, I believe we lose trust in both our bodies and our purpose. Finding the right doctor and moving towards improved physical health must be accompanied by the search to understand where our hearts want to serve. Swimming was a playground of sorts where the freedom to jump and splash provided self-expression and experimentation. I would later try painting, pottery, calligraphy—anything that got me making a mark and allowed me to see my self again.

Healing often begins when we engage with others. I had spent months living in a pink bathrobe. My walks in nature got me greeting strangers again. Meditating in a group setting became an important practice for me as well. What I enjoyed from these evening sessions was the sense of connection with others. Just knowing we had made time to be together, and were using this time to affirm our hope to live more compassionately, gave me greater courage. Finding a support group—and for me it really was a supportive vibration—can be very helpful.

Another pivotal group experience was an evening I spent with a women's drumming circle. I had never held a drum, nor thumped a deerskin hide. We began to beat in unison. As I slipped into the rhythm, I found myself filled with anxiety. It occurred to me I had been clinging so desperately to my past: to a body I once had, to a lover, to a career. Healing requires a willingness to accept, and to change. There would be a long period of rest before I would move with vigor or feel joy. The drumming circle helped me to understand that I needed to slow down. I needed to self-assess because the past I was clinging to was preventing me from making new decisions based on where I was now.

The swimming, the sickness, invited me to transcend the me of before, to join others in searching different dimensions of experience, sensation, and identity. I was more than my body, the broken physical structure that was slowly repairing. A circle of women rhythmically drumming had moved me farther out of the guilt and anxiety. My fall from an earlier path was not a failure, but an opening.

—Dana

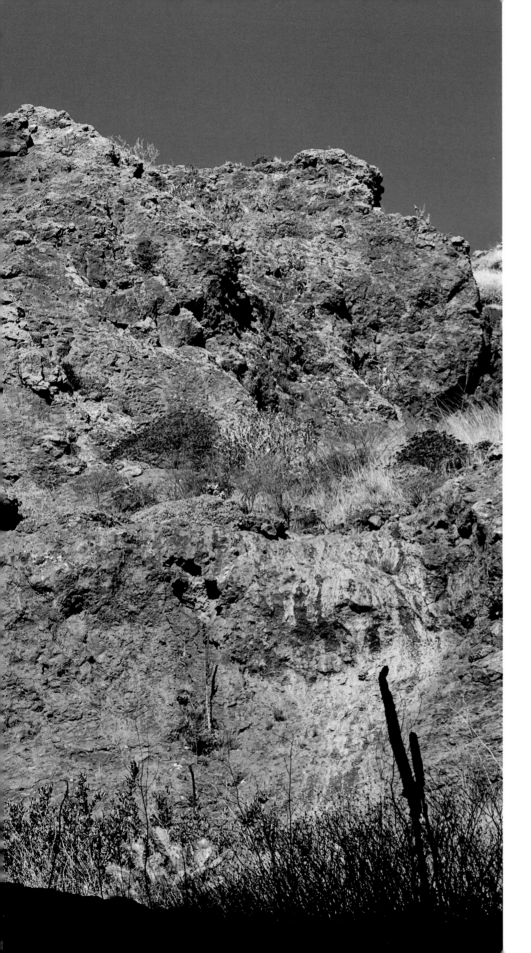

The Raven's Call
California

A Year of Transformative Work

The neurologist gave me a diagnosis that I didn't like, so I went to another, who word for word said the same thing: "There's no question about the diagnosis of multiple sclerosis, and we don't have any drugs for it yet." That was twenty years ago and I sought an alternative. I was fortunate to find the shamanic healing and empowerment group. Our leader had lived in South America with several tribes and honored their teachings and expected us to do the same. I joined a group process that would require monthly meetings for a year. The group became support for a select individual to prepare for a journey to the middle world, to the place of healing, personal and communal.

The "middle world" is not a continent or county. It is a place of new awareness, of different perspective. We didn't pretend to be shamans, but we learned much of their teachings of the ancient people, their sacred rituals, such as drumming and chanting. We took our journeys to discover what was out of balance in our personal lives or within our communities. The healing I felt was spiritual, solace in no longer feeling separation. I chose to be in nature instead of the fast-paced downtown of Wall Street. The imbalance in my life, I learned, was my separation from Earth and her creatures.

At first I was afraid, afraid that I no longer belonged to my society, that I was giving up what I had fought and worked for. My idea of fulfillment was askew. If money didn't buy health and happiness, then what was the purpose of work? Native people offered a spiritual reality different from mine, where trees are divine and power animals are guides. Balance is key, as is giving back and caring for the spirits in all beings. During my afternoon walk from my home, a raven dove down from a tree, reminding me of the many worlds, haunting and exalted, that many of us ignore. The experience made me realize I wouldn't go back again to that other life. Ravens are the spirit carriers in some tribes, animals that mediate between life and death. For me, they carried away my sickness, the sickness of separation.

I walked softly on the earth. I felt the rhythms of the seasons in my body, was glad for the break of day over the land where I lived. I passed time not needing entertainment or even comradeship except for the birds and my dog. I didn't feel trapped in my body; rather, I learned to feel gratitude for it, even with its quirks and refusal to respond to my wishes. I began to realize my body was the container for my spirit that travelled away when I drummed with the shamanic group. The handicaps of my disease that had forced me to change my life so drastically also were rewards. I was released to explore other sides of myself, forced to embrace a new understanding of wholeness and accept that I am connected to all things, that my physical being is only a part of me. My trials for success in the financial world, which had been my only reference, were no longer relevant.

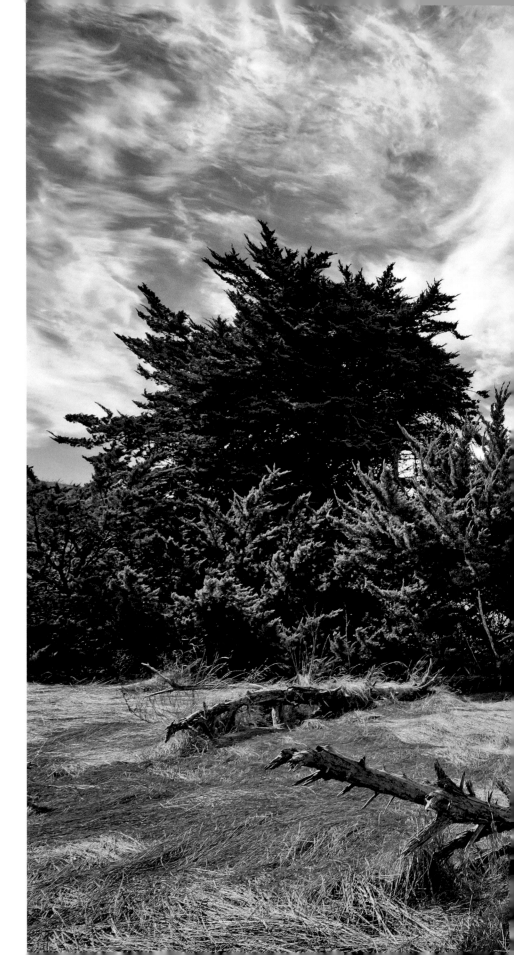

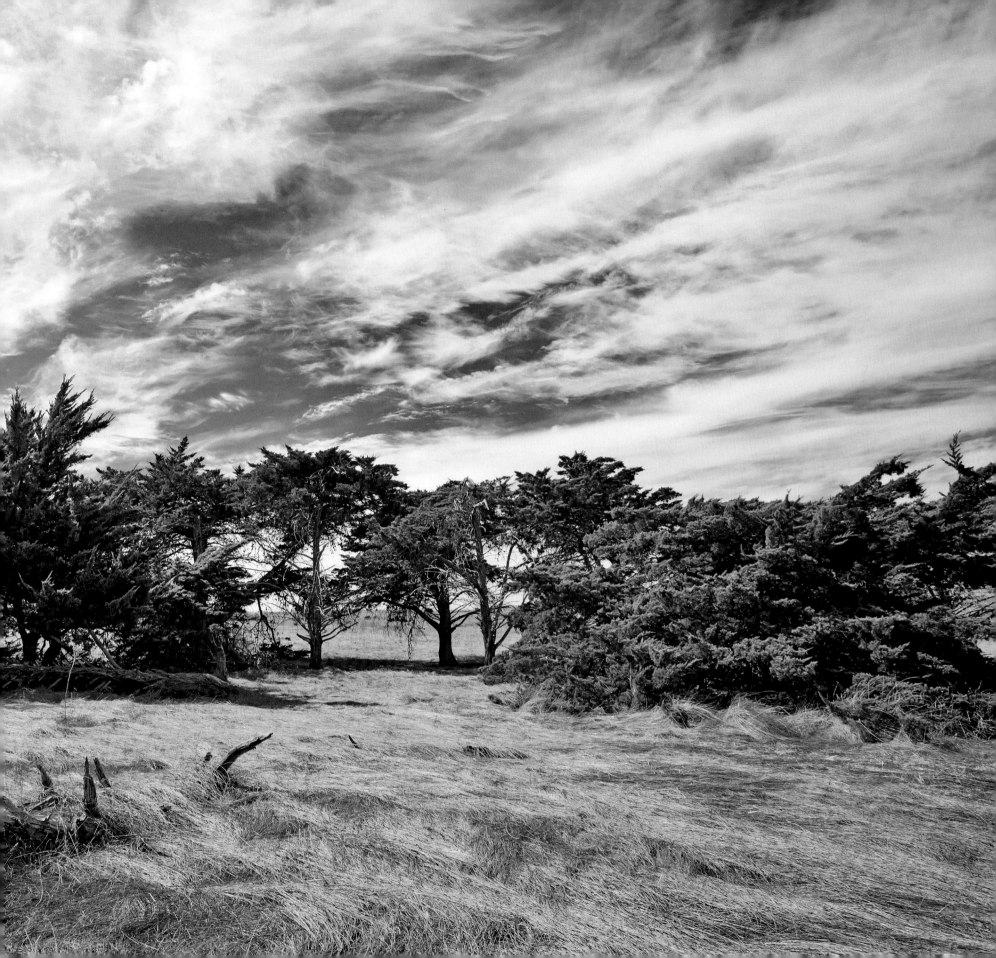

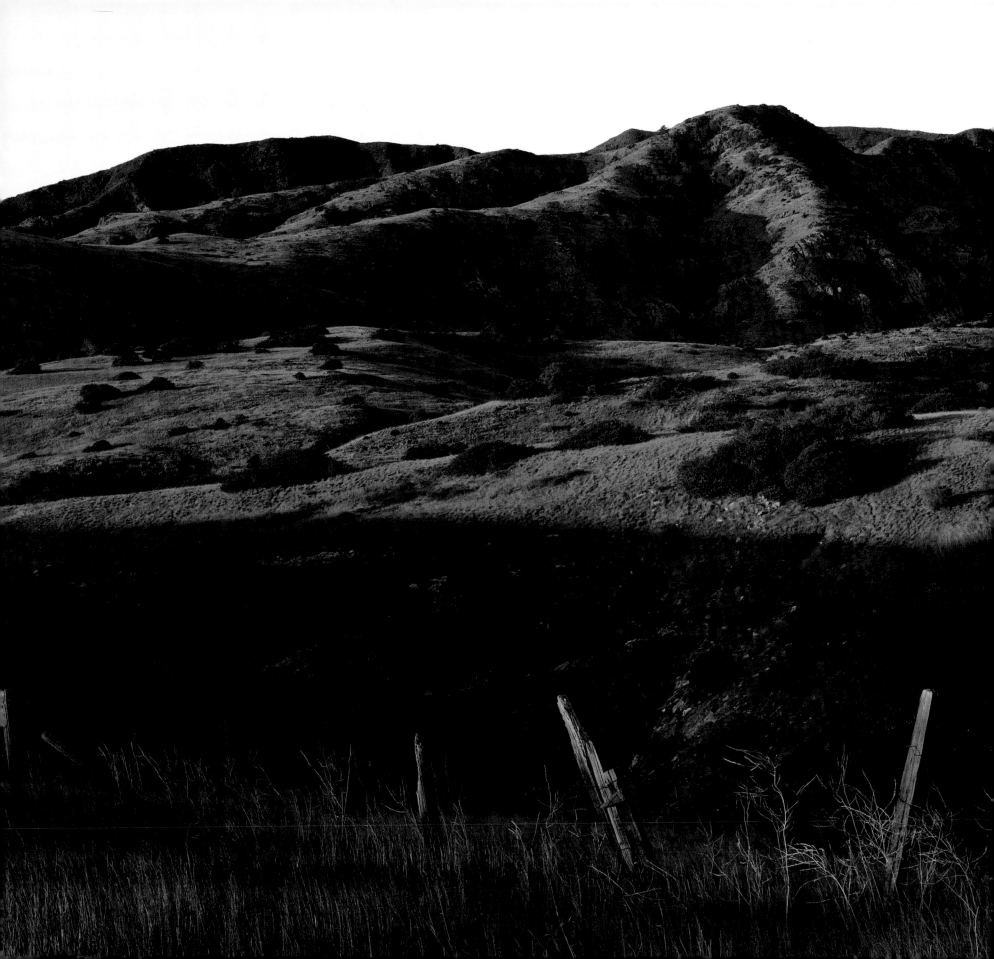

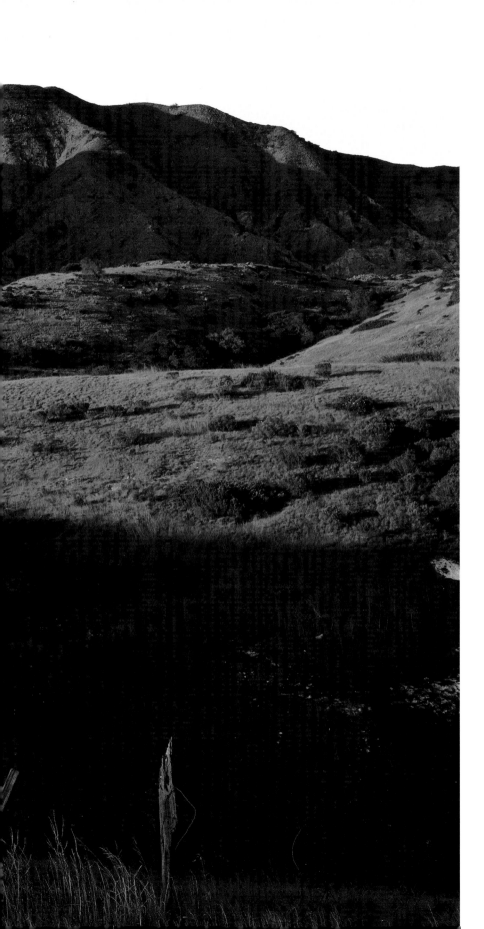

The other members of my group provided a deeper bond than I had ever known, in spite of my seeing them only once a month. We came out of our egos when one of us held "the talking stick," sharing intentions for the time ahead in preparation for journeying to the other world the following month. This year of shamanic ritual was very different for all of us who had come from a business life of competition in cities across the country, where each day we walked on soiled pavement to the chaotic sounds of traffic. Birdsong and silence were childhood memories that I chose as companions during this period of healing. I emerged from my year with a sense of inner peace and balance and a profound sense of union with the natural world. I would lie on the Earth and feel her strength and give my gratitude. Decades of scurrying to fulfill dubious achievements were now in the past.

—Karen

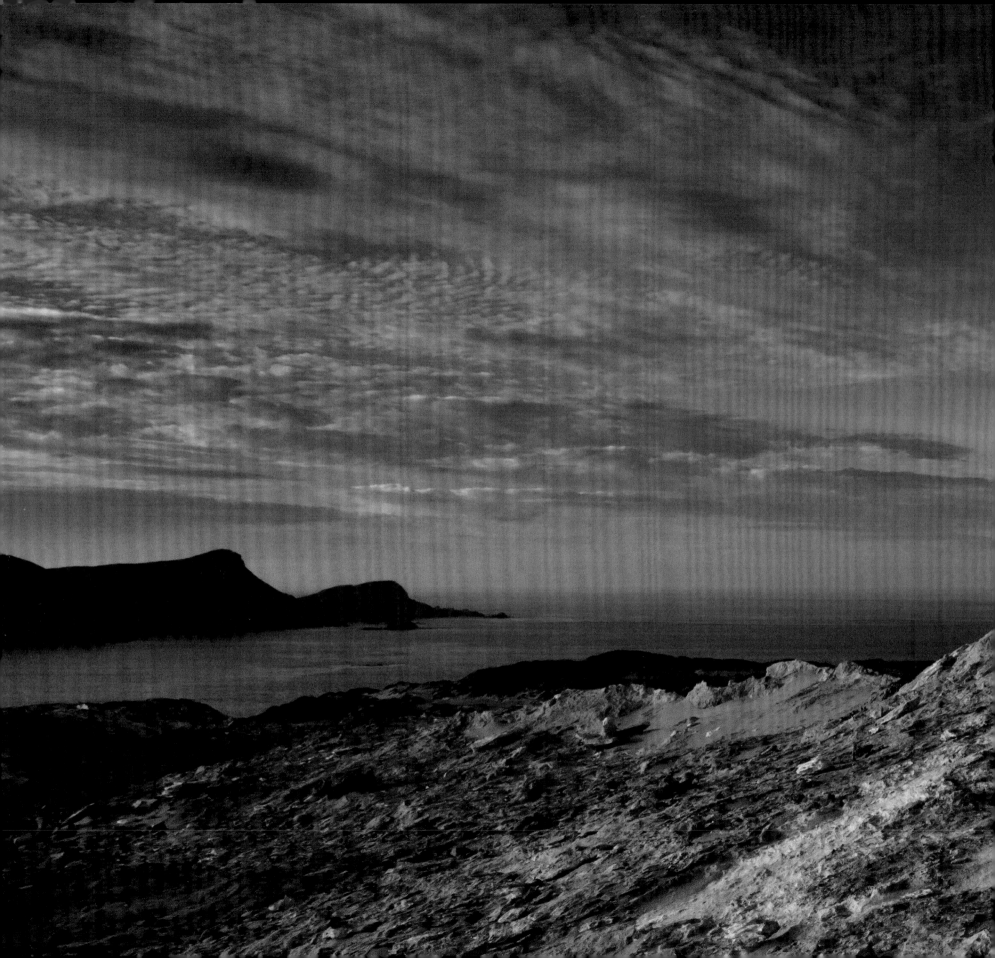

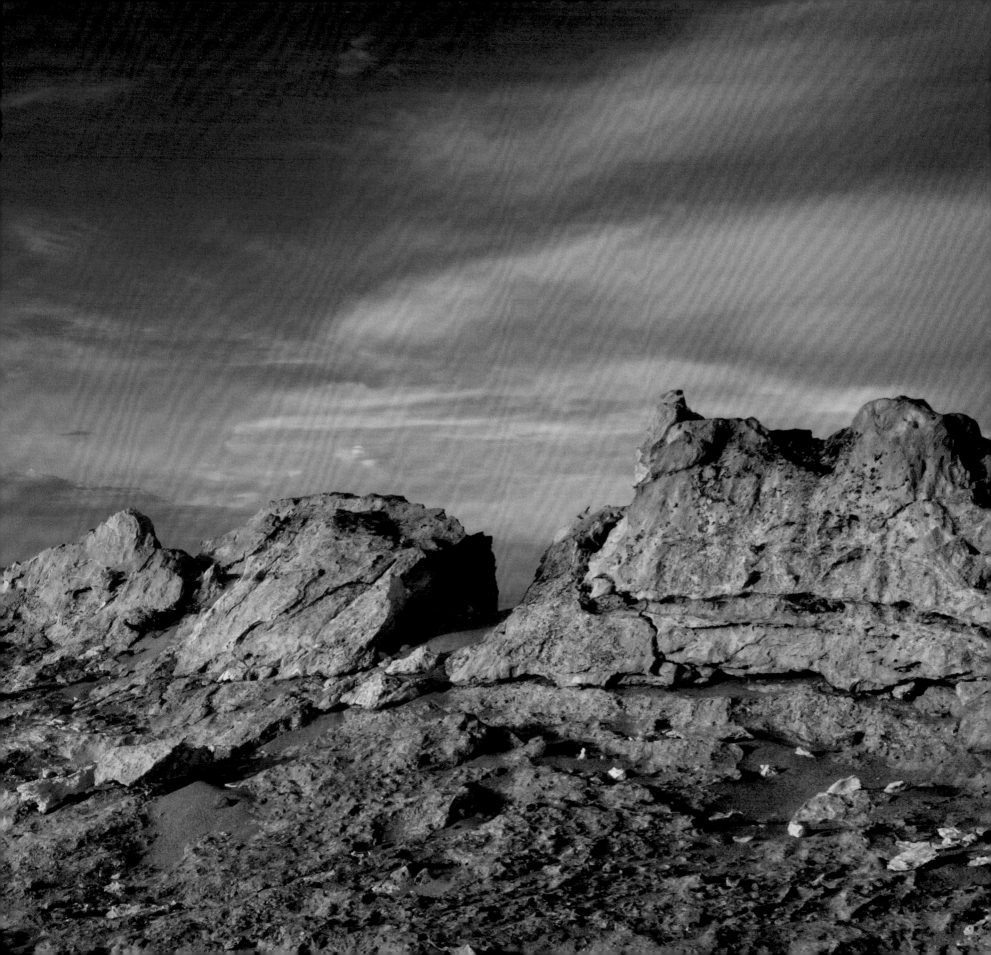

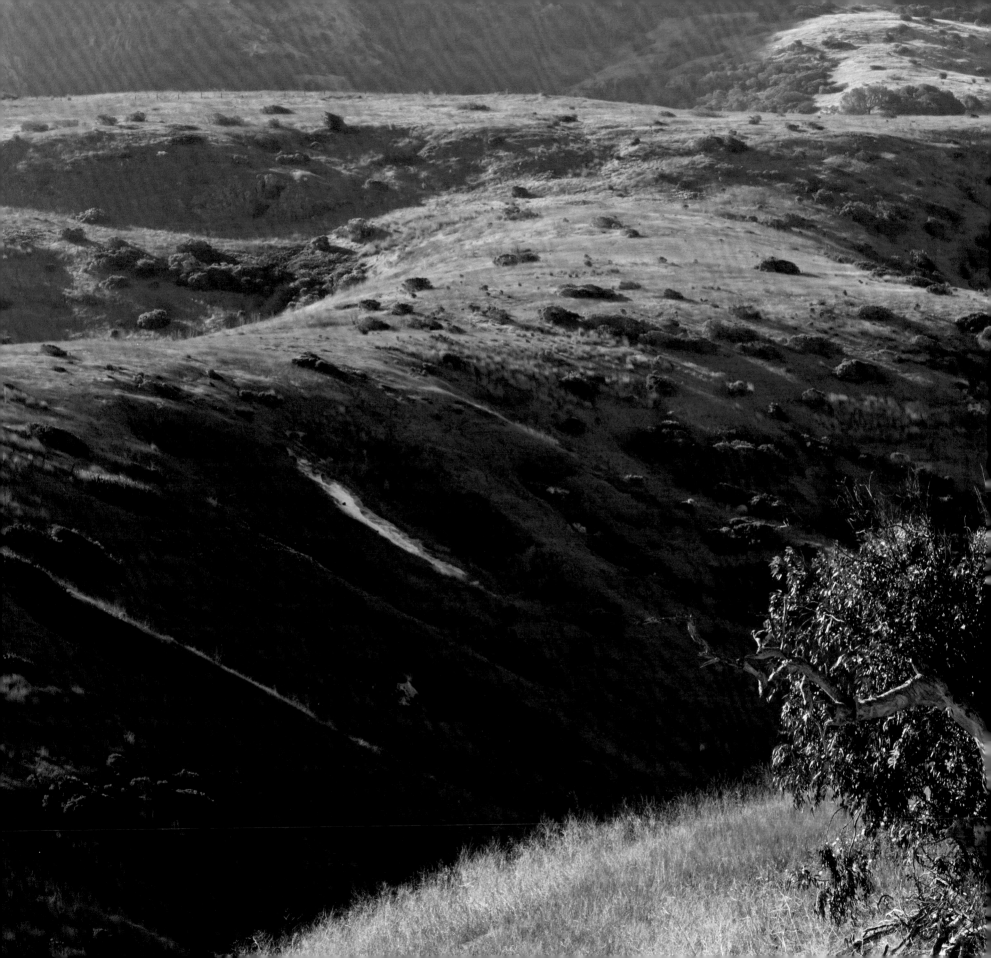

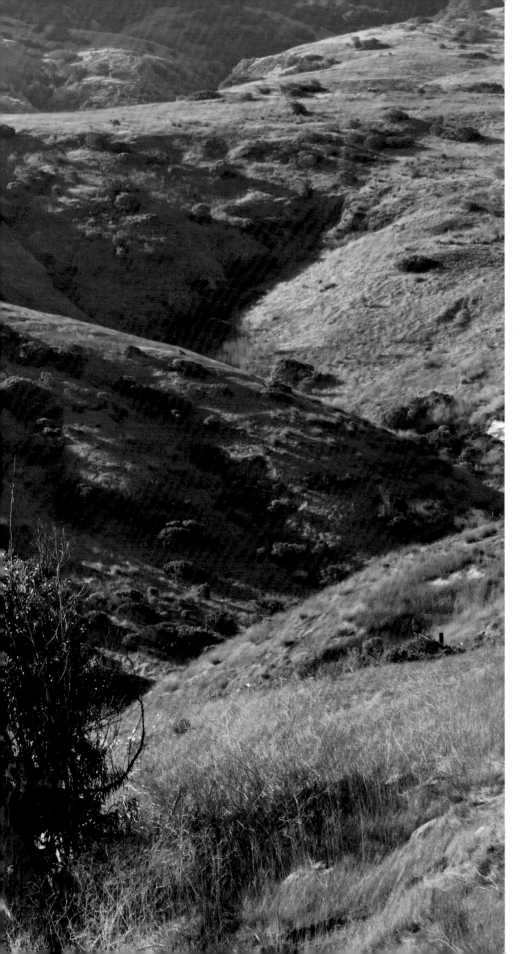

Singing the Voice Within

I felt unprepared to be in the presence of a healing elder. Perhaps I had never truly believed. Or, perhaps, the limits of my ego were slipping away as I responded to a man who clearly possessed sacred wisdom. There were voices in his world, invisible spirits and guides. Sometimes we need to walk with these elders to find our way back to ourselves.

His name is Angaangaq Angakkorsuaq, and he is from Greenland. I was standing alone with him in a small room in a Southern California home. He began drumming, then chanting. His voice was powerful, uncanny, yet embracing. With eyes closed, I felt myself sway. I knew I had to dig into myself and stand tall. My journey began in the water, moving under his current of sound. I moved onto land and felt my feet root into the earth. Finally, I soared in the great sky.

He continued to circle me in step and sound. I was swept up in the deep bellows of his voice, as his chant intensified into the roar of a mountain lion. I felt as if I had unlocked a door and was confronted with my deepest fears. The darkness inside moved in a spiral, becoming a cyclone—then left my body. I felt more and more connected to my inner strength the more I listened to my elder. His voice contained every season, every essence! In the final moments of our session, I heard my voice slowly rise to join his. My own little voice was being "called" out of me. I wept tears of love for the tender singing I heard from within. It was timid and childlike, and waiting to be born.

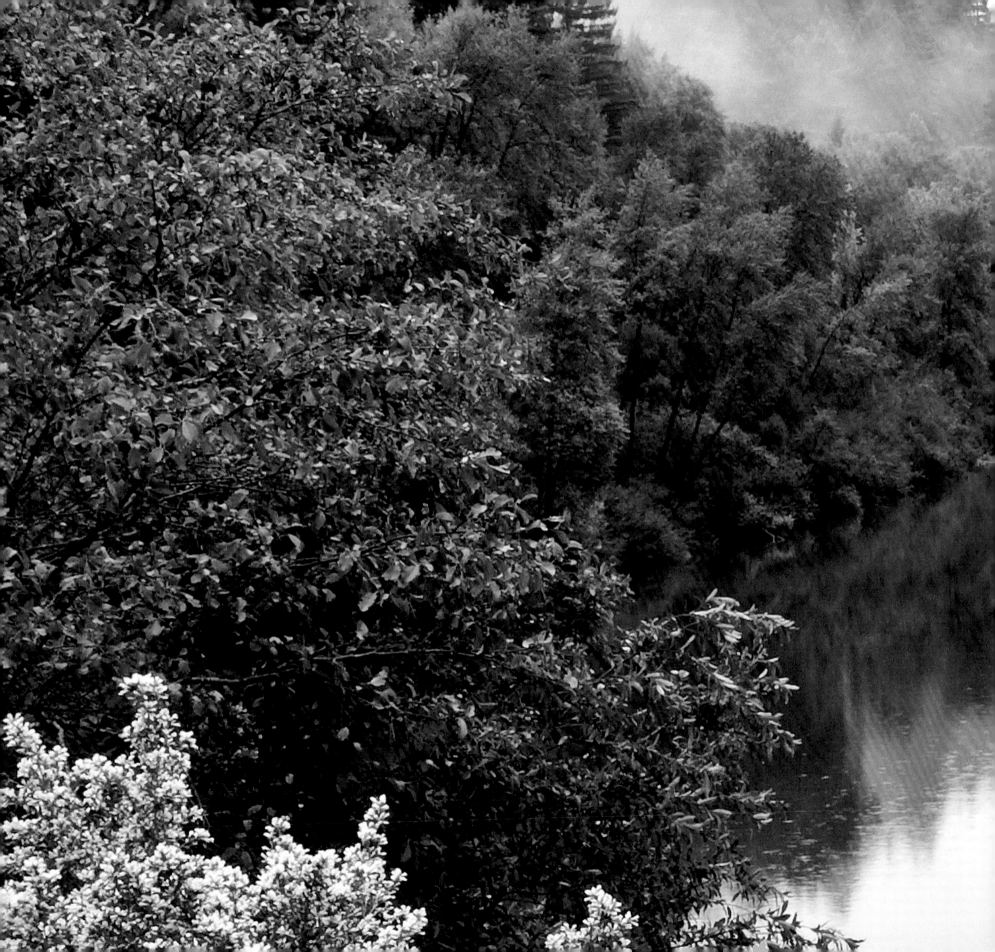

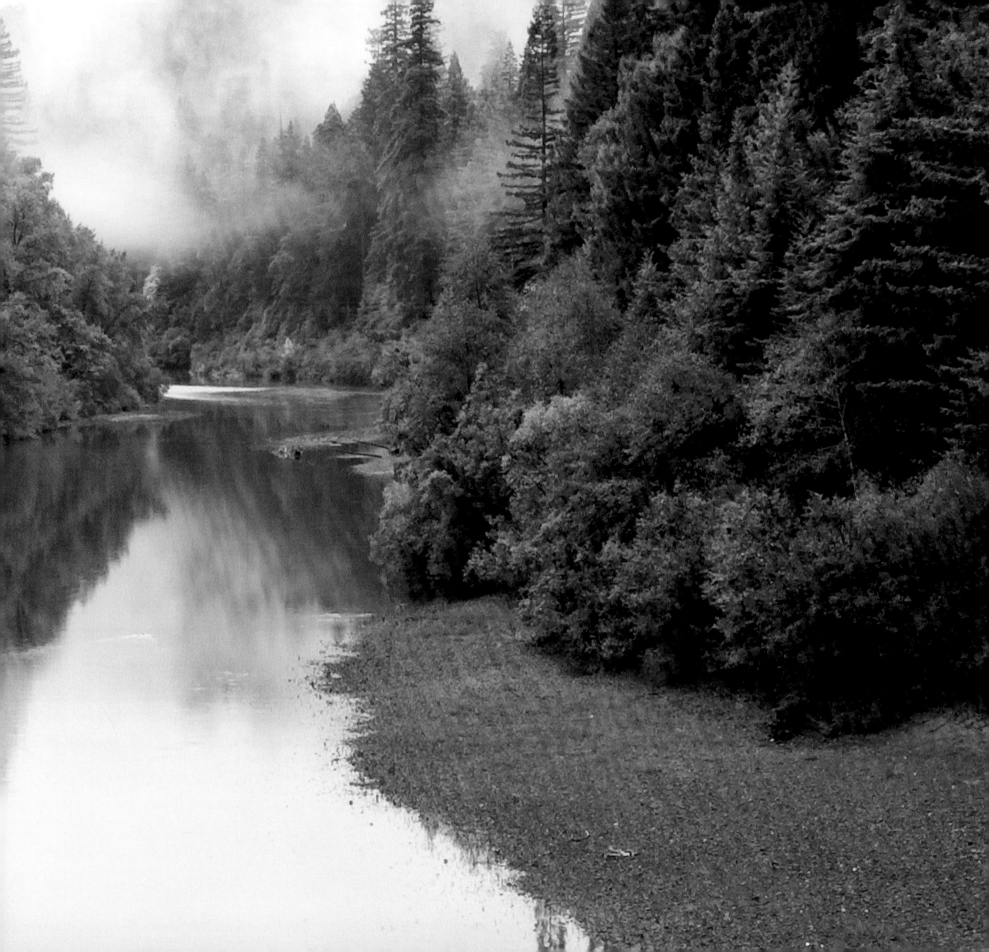

As I drove away, I was filled with laughter. The laughter seemed to loosen the shackles of a false belief. I could no longer see separation between myself and the people around me. The traffic light, representing all the rules we choose to follow, made me aware that we each accept the beliefs that structure our view of the world. My laughter shifted my perspective, showing me the infinite possibilities that exist in every moment. I felt an all-encompassing love for all of creation. As the boundaries between my self and the world began to dissolve, a sense of peace surrounded me. If we share one consciousness, nothing needs to limit our experiences. I may have been daydreaming in a new self-awareness, but I was profoundly inspired to imagine a healed body, a more enlivened spirit, a connected consciousness.

—Dana

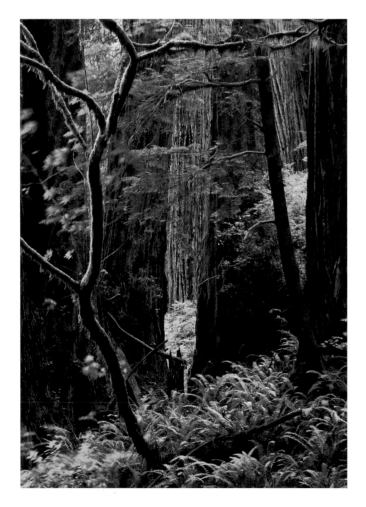

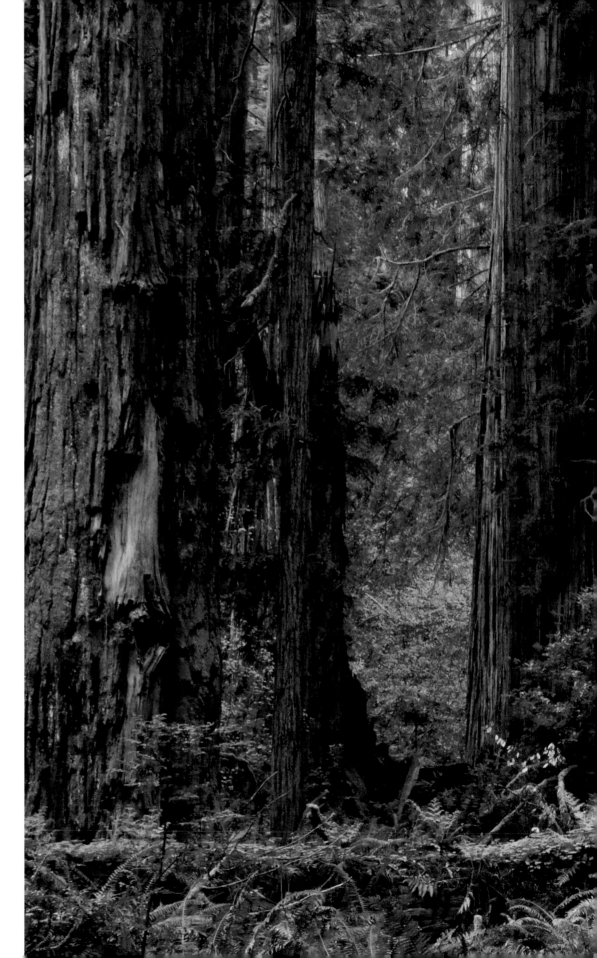

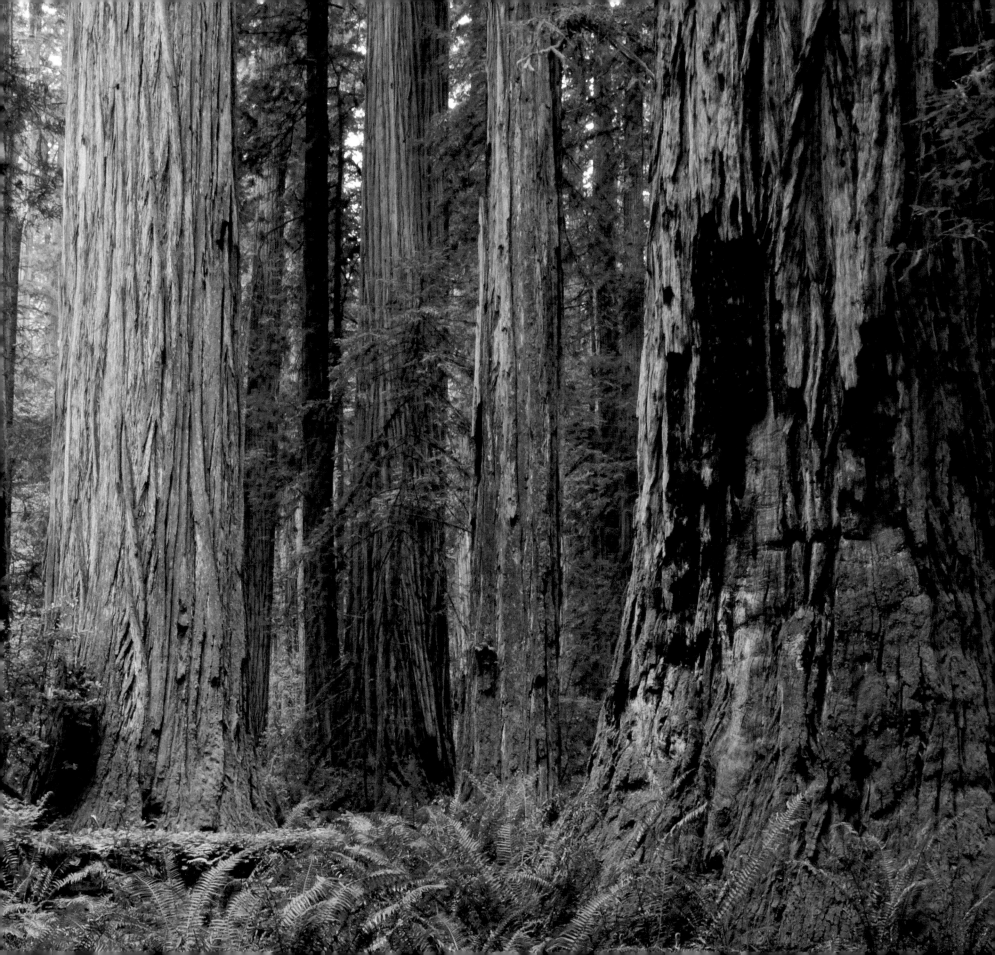

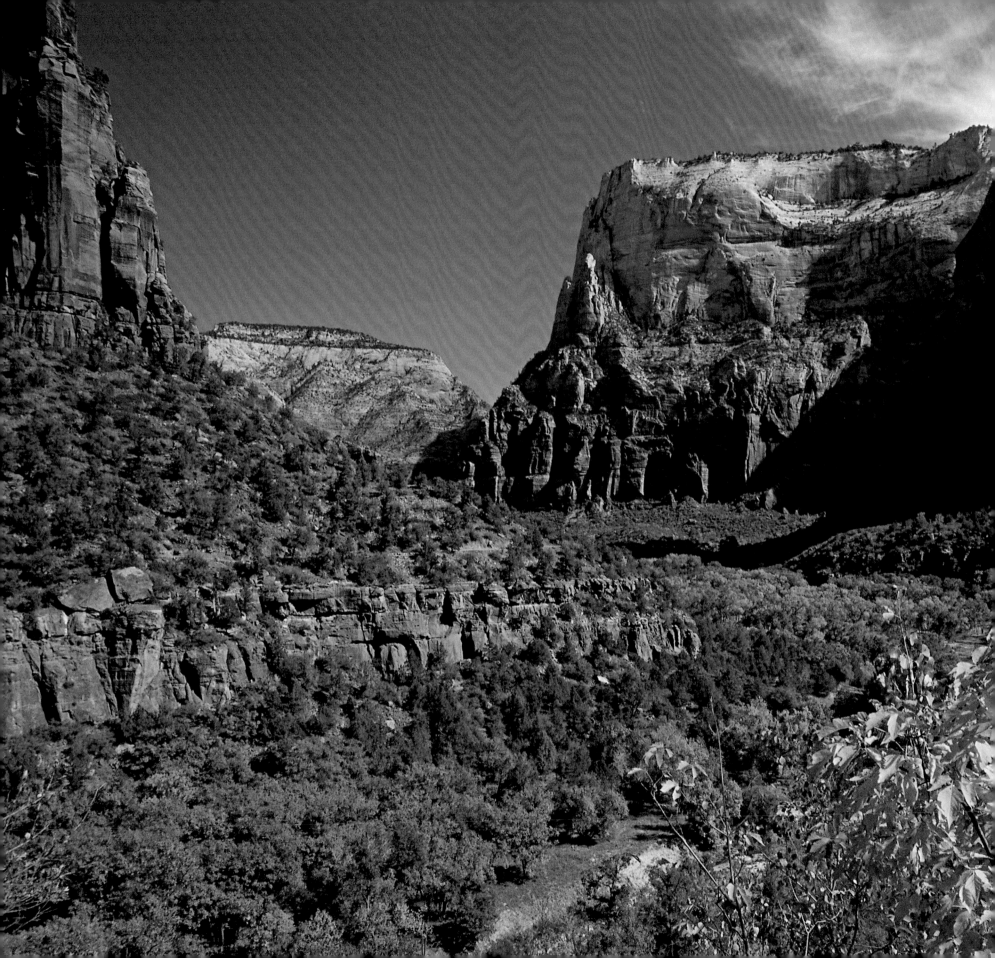

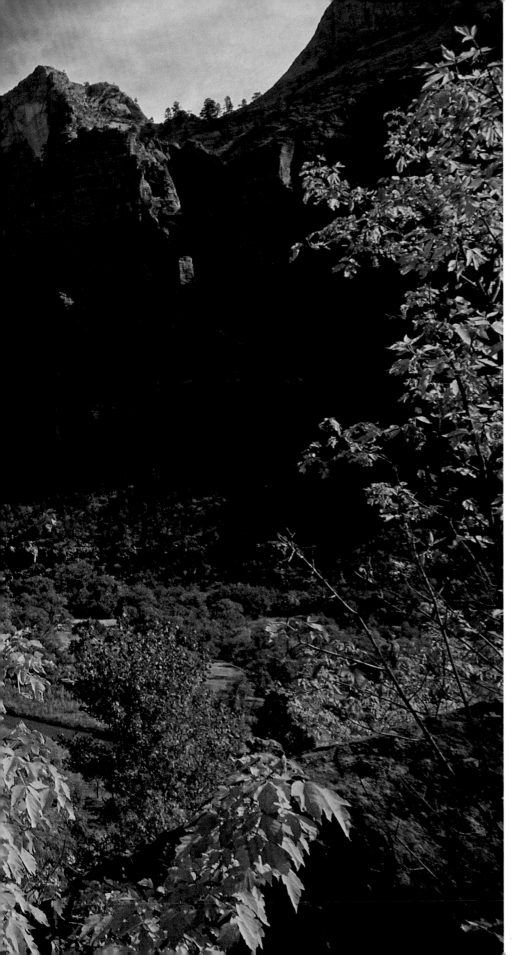

Being Guided
Zion, Utah

This is a place where you walk between cracks in the earth. Canyons fissured by water and wind rise beside you. Erosion has built this place—a sanctuary of red sand. Sunlight and shadows move across the rocks and beckon to invisible forces that carved these rock faces. Some see the hand of the Maker; others explain with words of geology. Oh, how to describe these skyscraping monoliths!

For ten hours, my companion and I would crisscross the Virgin River during a sixteen-mile trek down The Narrows of Zion. A one-hour drive brought us to cow pastures and forests of ponderosa pines. Along a dirt path we began, passing an abandoned cabin and tools turning to rust. Hand-sawed logs interlocked against wind and rain, day and night.

The sound of water brought us into a ravine where a short crossing invited me to practice rock hopping. With eyes downcast, I leaped. Perhaps my restricted view, blocked by the brim of my baseball cap, had emboldened me to jump farther and higher; however, it came with a consequence. A tree had fallen and now rested above. Sailing for a moment, I suddenly collided with the trunk I never saw. Terror swept over me. Everything in my body asked the same question: Is my neck broken?

Hesitantly, I leaned forward, turned and stretched, discovering only tightness. The headache began. For the rest of our walk, I would rely on my partner to do the neck bending to reveal the sights above. Much of my experience that afternoon came from his words and imagination. He revealed the poetry of the place in perceptions I had not heard from him before.

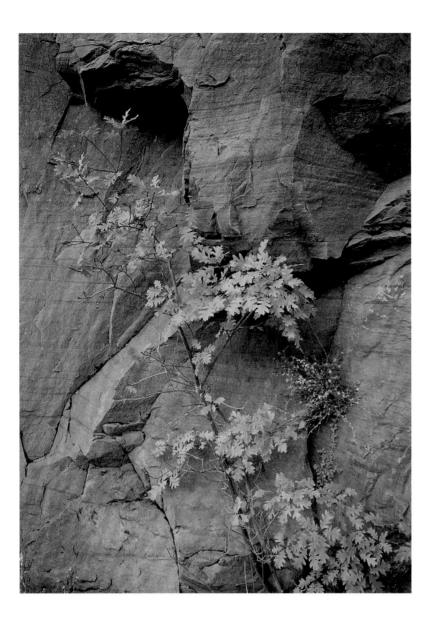

Our route depended on water depth, sections of sandy streambed, and available high ground. I followed the hundreds of decisions my partner made that day. As I walked, I thought about our connection, about the path we were creating and the interpersonal journey. Relationships "let the light in" and expose fundamental beliefs we have held like bedrock. Learning to share our values, insecurities, and dreams is an endless, rewarding assessment of who we are becoming. I realized this landscape of shifting sand had become my inner world as well. Our hands leaned on canyon walls as water parted beneath our feet.

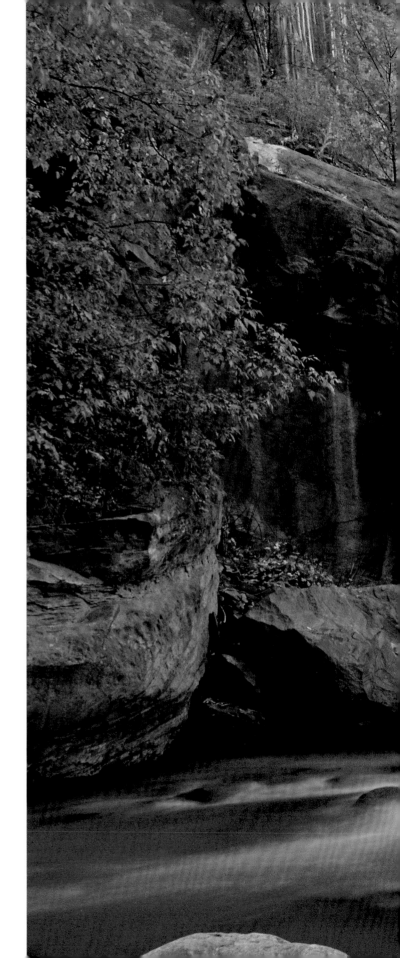

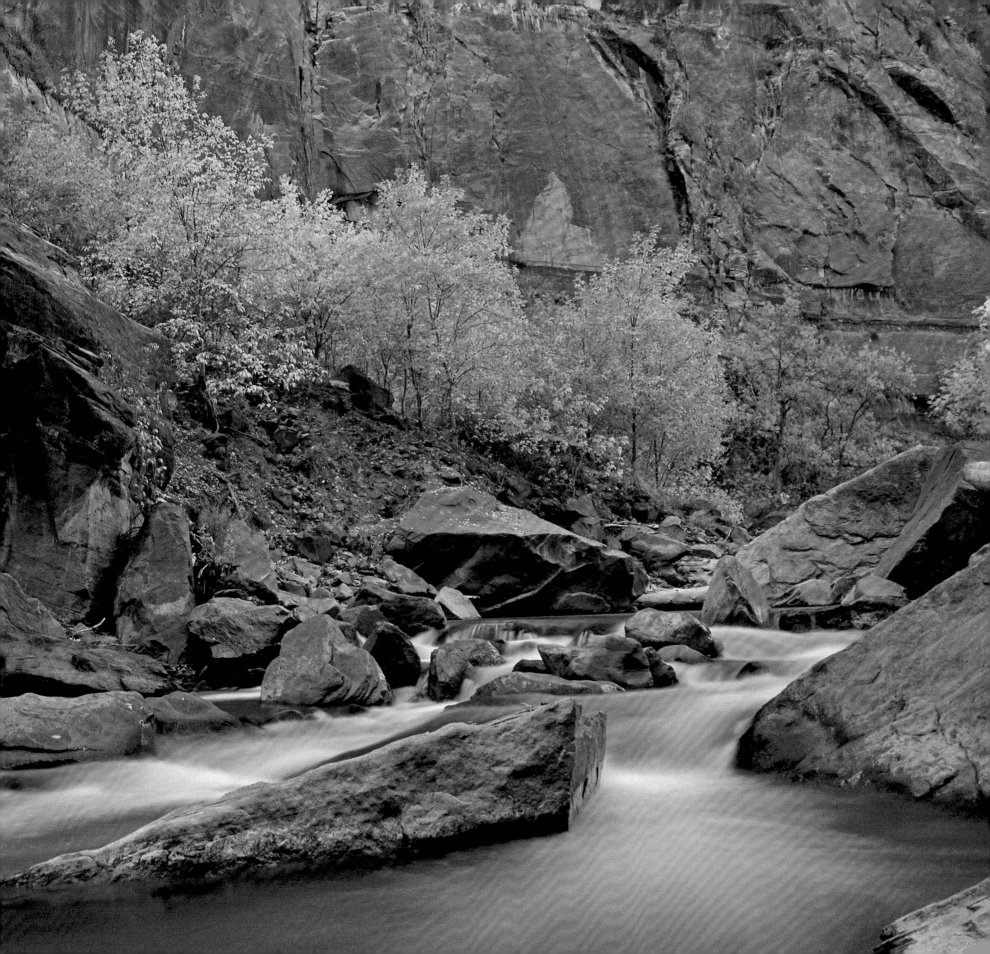

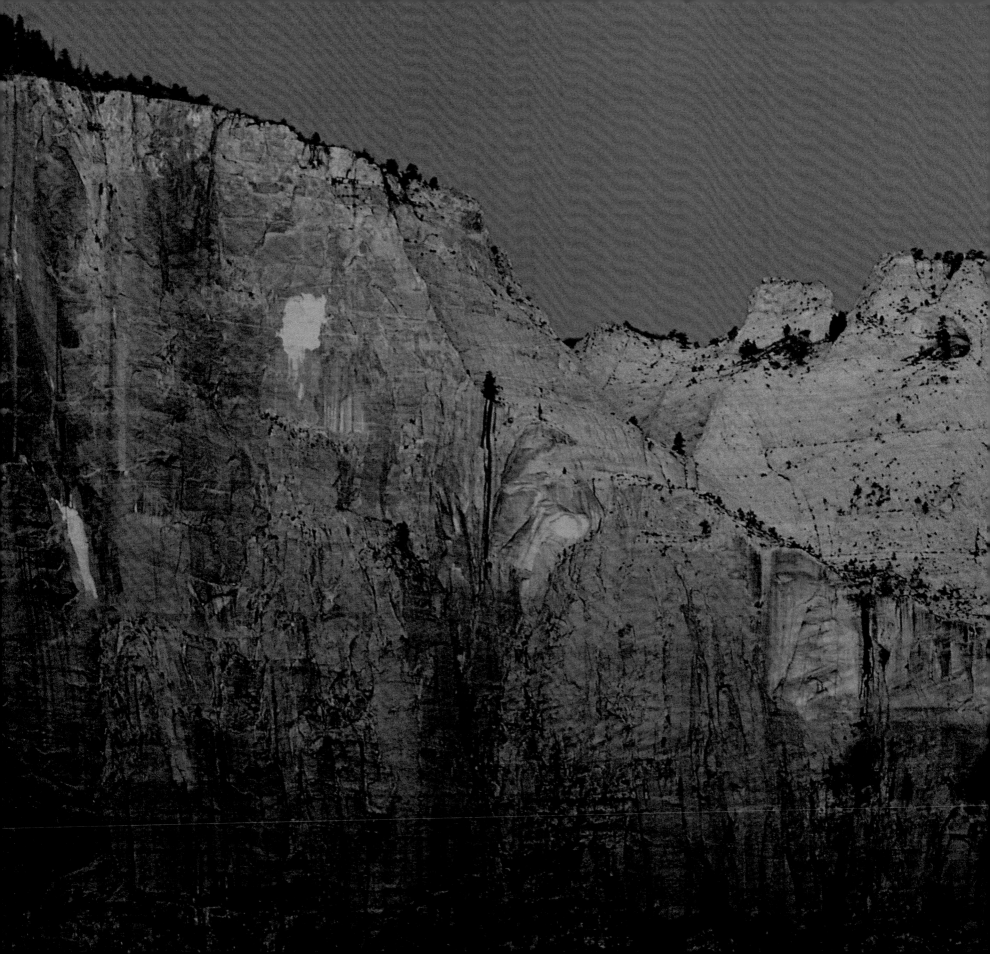

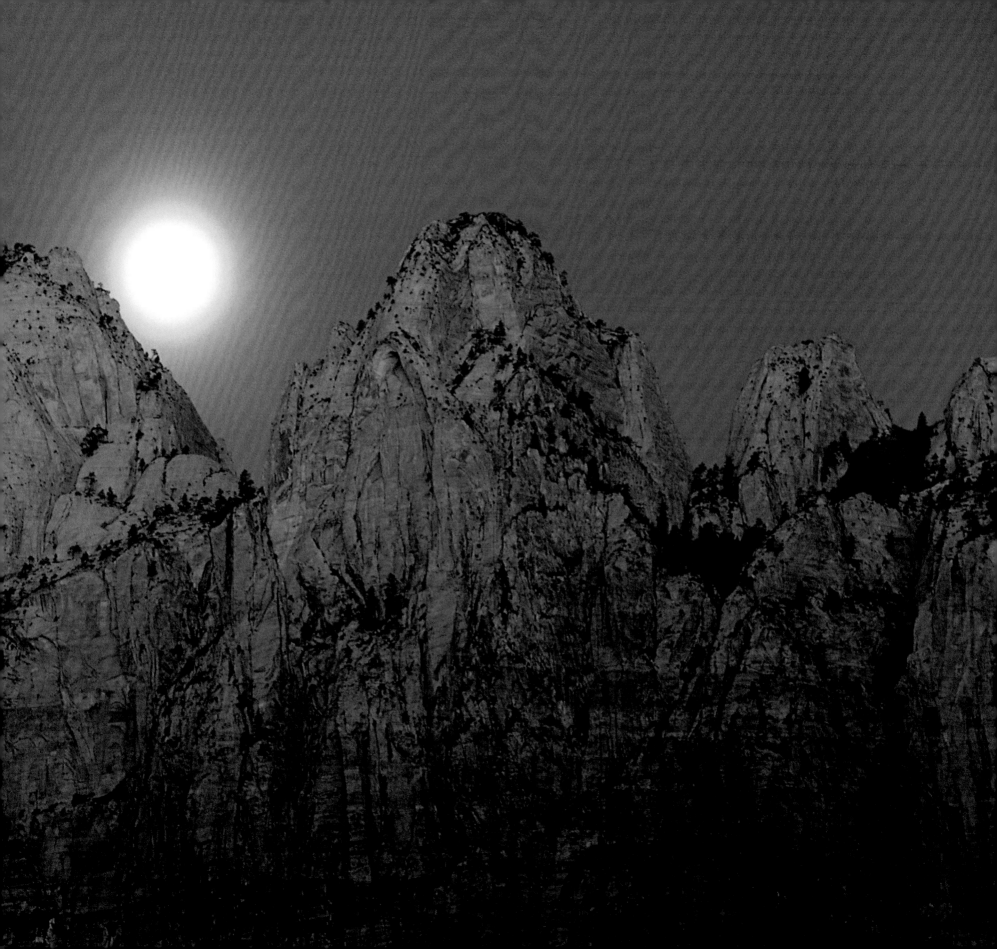

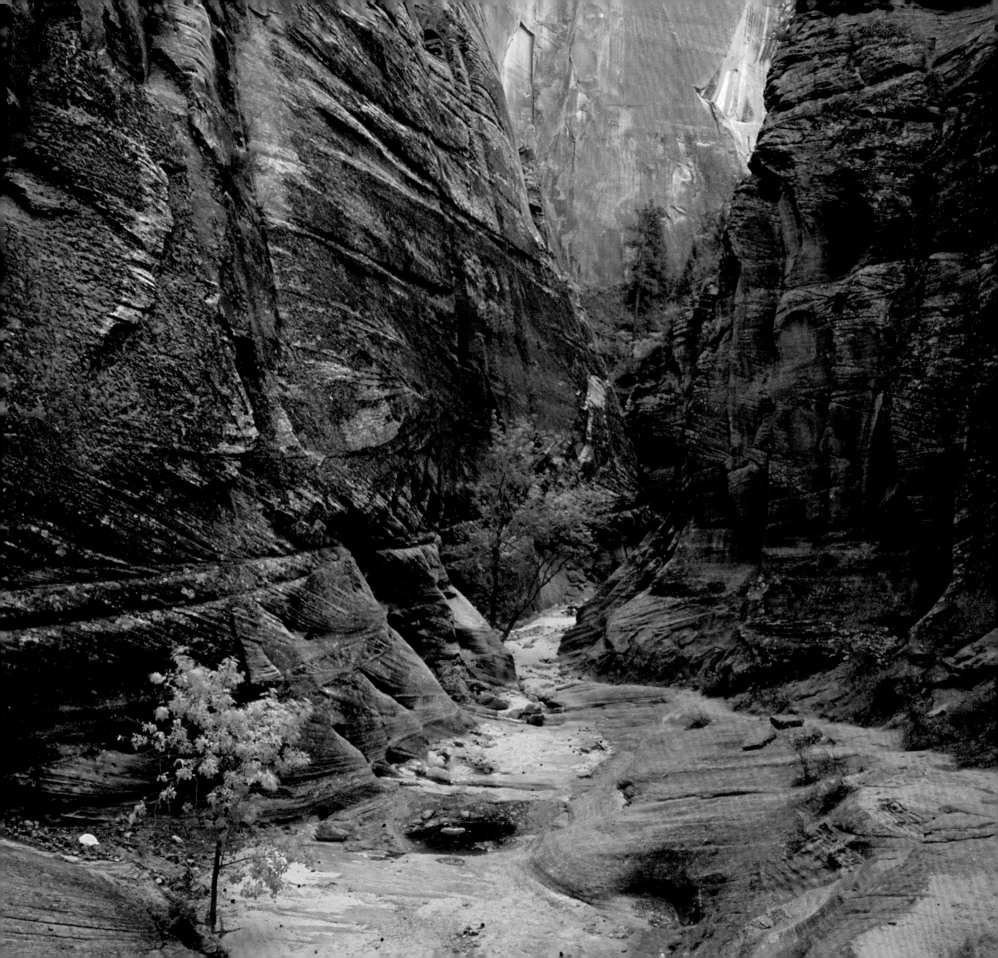

My steps were timid, but water caught me each time I slipped. Pacing was critical, and I focused on learning the right distance to follow. Proximity to my partner was necessary to observe the course and steer clear of unsteady surfaces, but keeping some space between us was equally important to allow pause and redirection. Decision making moved between collaboration and independence.

Over high ledges, hanging gardens of fern and moss reached for sunlight above. Birds floated into the narrow stretch of rock through which we passed, finding a small cave or peak to rest. A sudden streak of silver at our feet reminded us of the fish below. We carried a map, which identified the creeks that crossed this section of river. Holding this guide at the bottom of the canyon, I could only imagine the land above. In The Narrows, where we walked, progress could not be tethered to a landmark growing in clarity. Progress was made one step at a time. The rush of water from a side canyon carried sediment from an unknown territory. We waded through this confluence, sensing something of our selves was also being carried away.

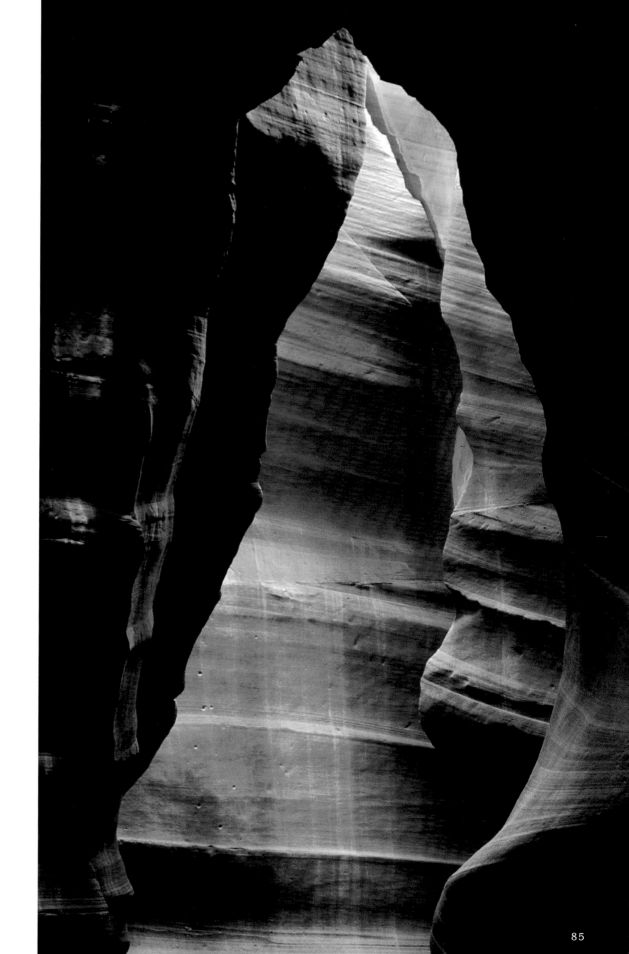

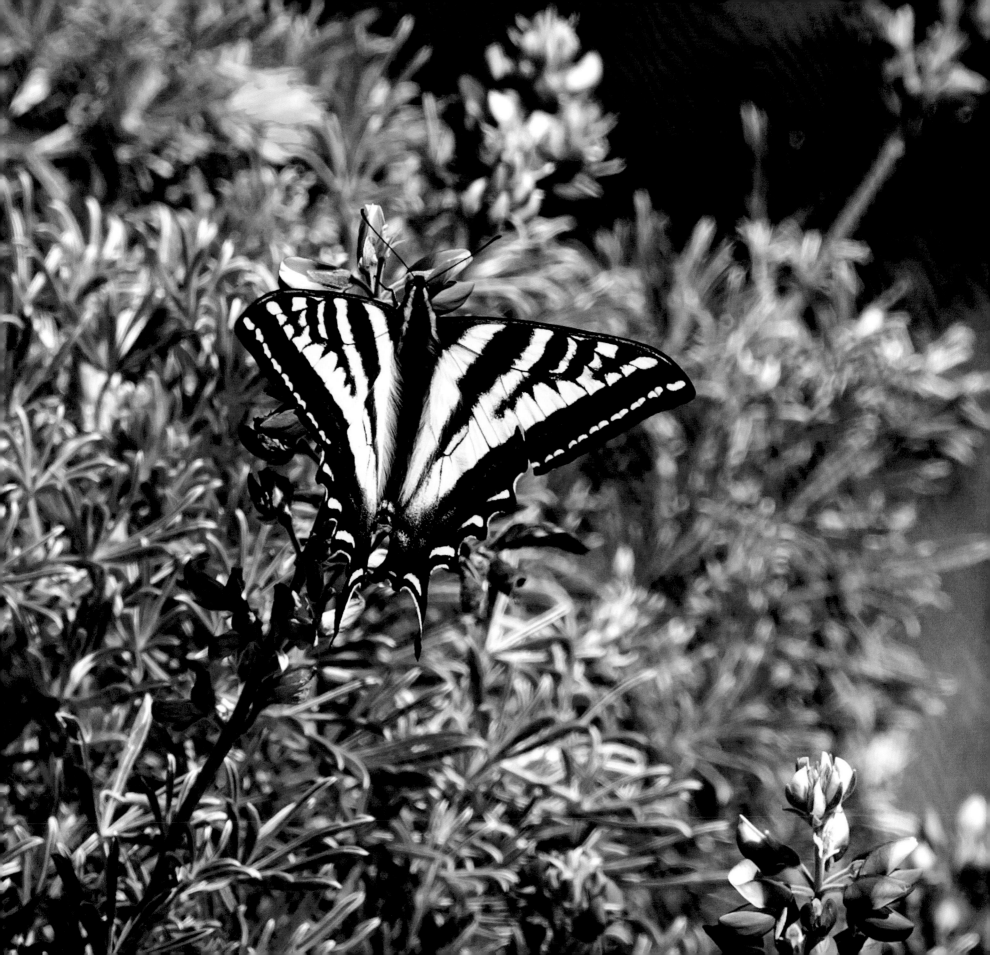

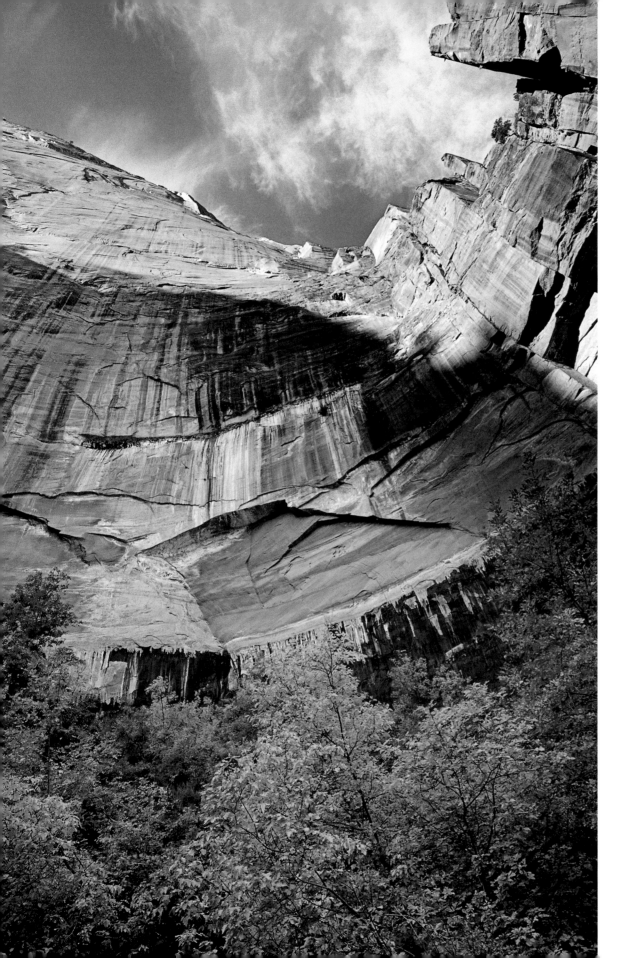

Meeting people approaching from upstream was like encounters with explorers on voyages of discovery. Each of us had questions for the other: What is it like where you have been? How much farther? Such interactions were surprisingly welcome after hours of isolation. We appreciated the infrequency of visitors, but each time we passed, it seemed to reassure us we were not lost. People come into our lives to help us find our way.

Our final afternoon in Zion National Park was spent hiking the gradual curve of a mountain slope. We rested in the shade of a tree, stretching our bodies over the smooth rock, hands entwined. We listened to the wind as it swept across our skin and clothing. There was music. My partner expressed concern about my fear of hurting myself. It was true I had needed continual consolation after hitting my head. For him, my reaction was isolating. He compared it to watching me disappear on a precipice he could not reach. Was he asking for trust? Did he hope to reassure me when I felt overwhelmed and uncertain? A black and yellow butterfly circled us several times. My mind seemed to open to the insect's freedom and the dance of a zigzag. I had turned away from intimacy for so many years. It was time to take another leap through the gates of Zion.

—Dana

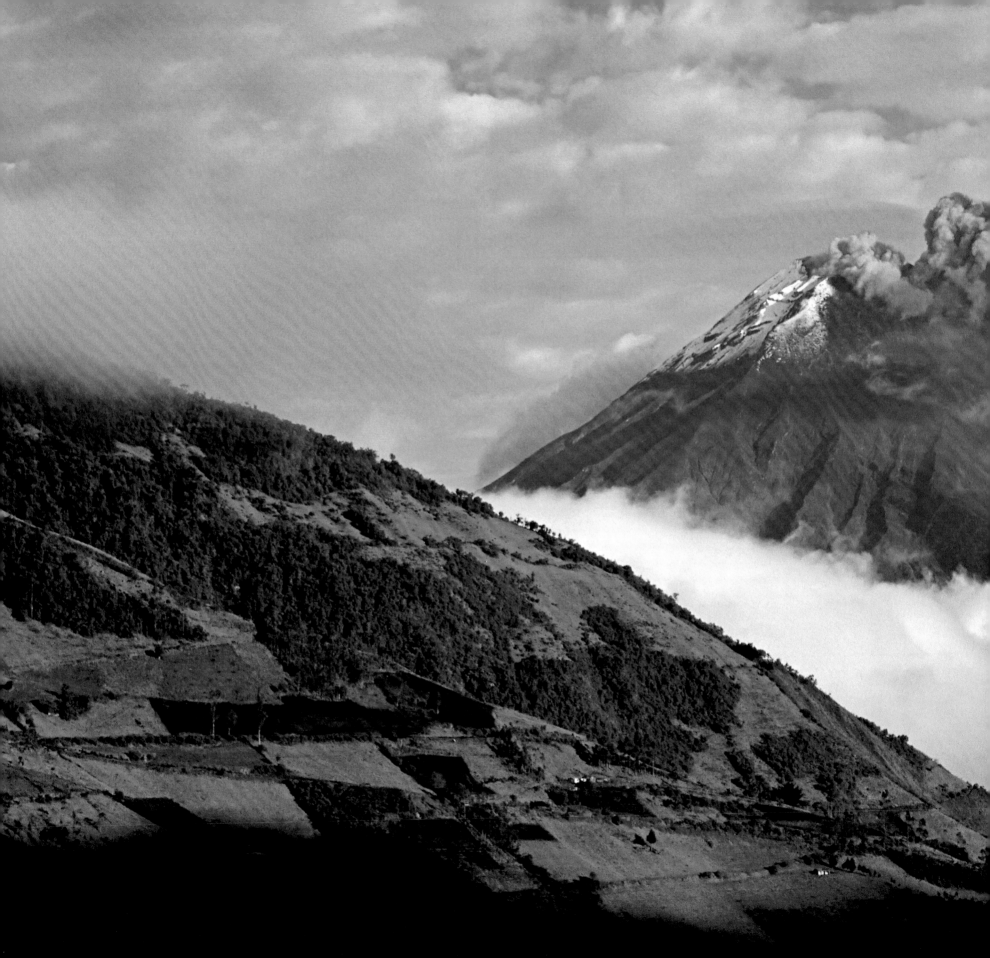

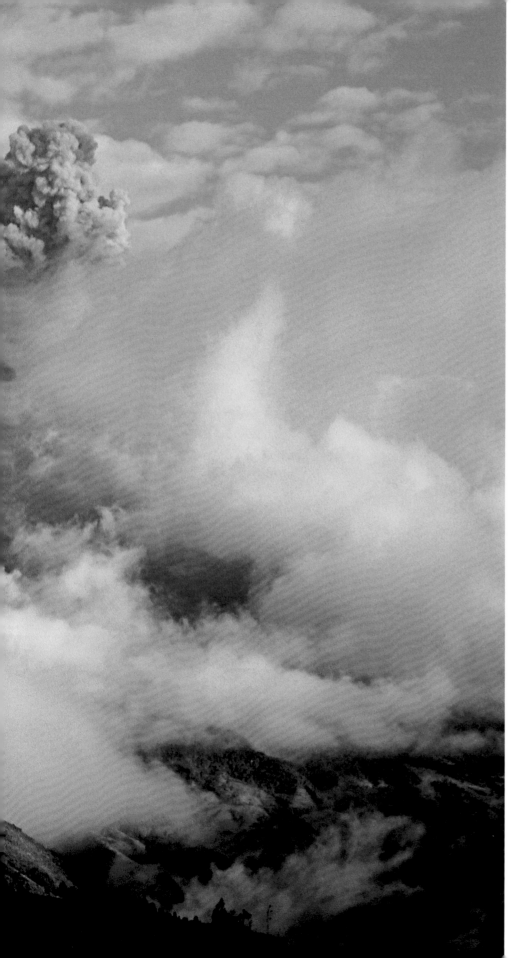

Cloud Forest
Ecuador

Under a canopy of leaf in the waves of birdsong, I enter the cloud forest. It is here where spires of green hold up the sky and moisture is pulled from clouds to jungle floor. In this forest, my body surrenders to the nourishment of moist air and dappled light.

There is a simple lodge where hummingbirds abound. Feeders are hung on trees most everywhere to keep the busy birds returning. Despite this abundance of pink sugar water, the hummingbirds are quick to chase each other. I watch the intricate, sometimes fierce, battles and wonder if these birds have stopped searching for the wildflowers. With such diversity in plant and animal species, what does it mean to drink from a plastic feeder? Does the hummingbird still marvel at the delicate petals and, in the stillness of his beating wings, extend a beak down the curved lip of a fragrant blossom?

The cloud forests of the Andes are among the richest in the world biologically, and among the least understood. Thousands of flowers affirm so many ways to thrive, yet it is predicted that Ecuador will be completely deforested in thirty years.

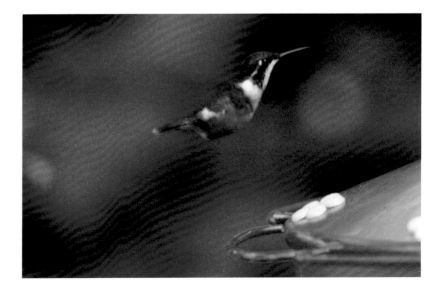

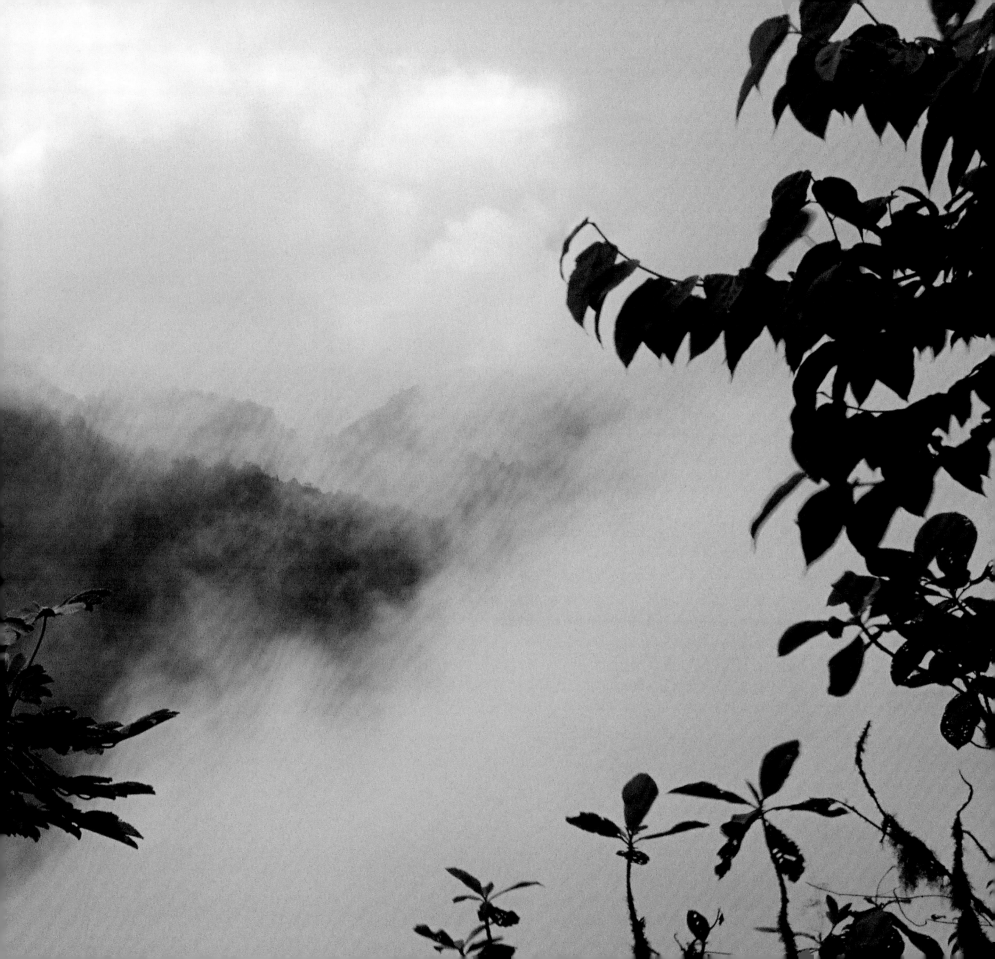

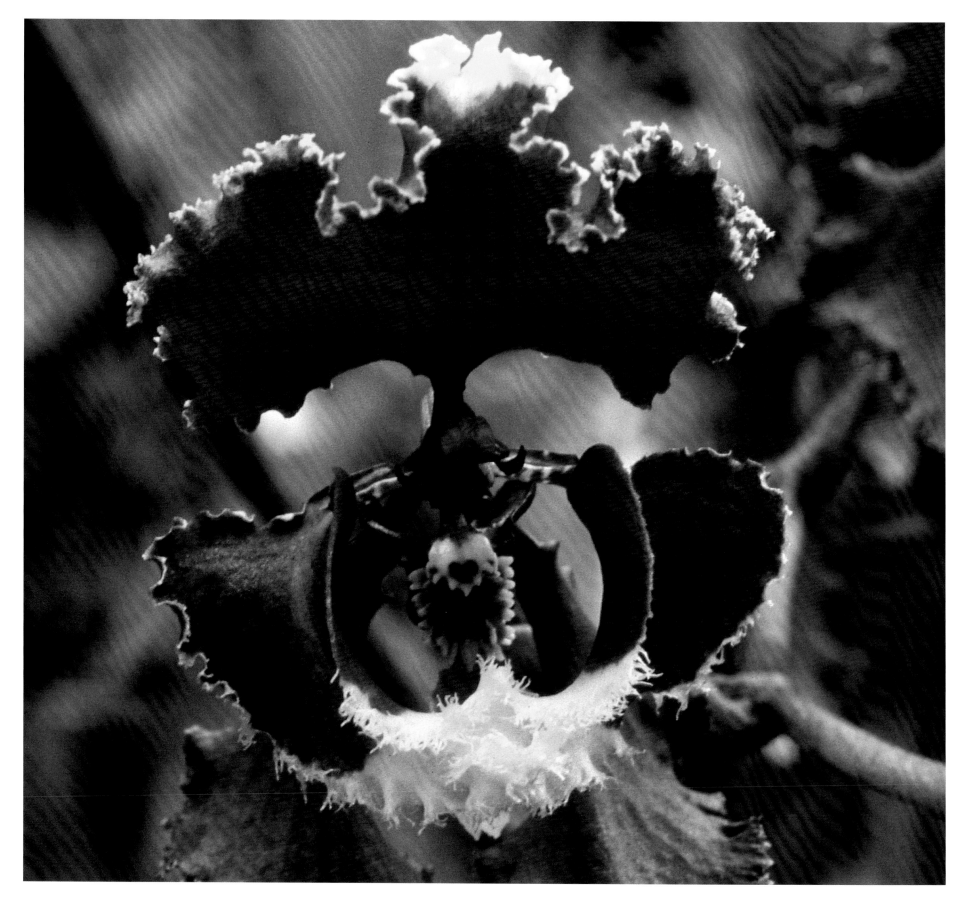

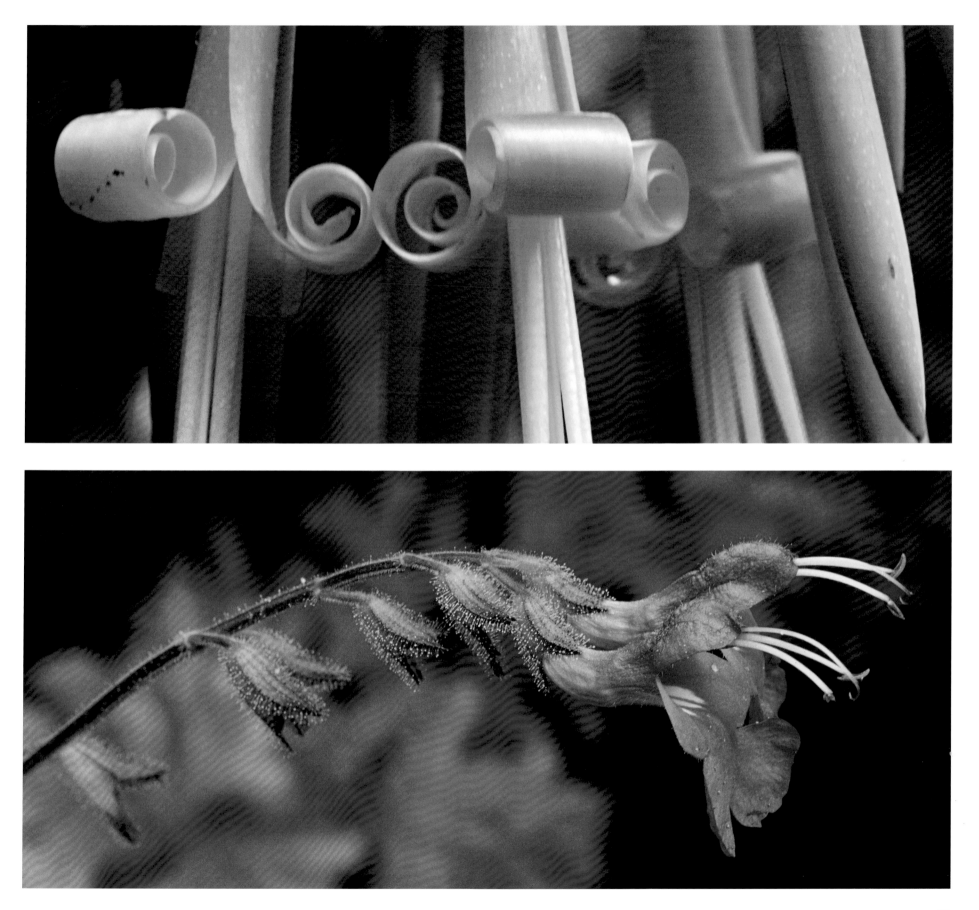

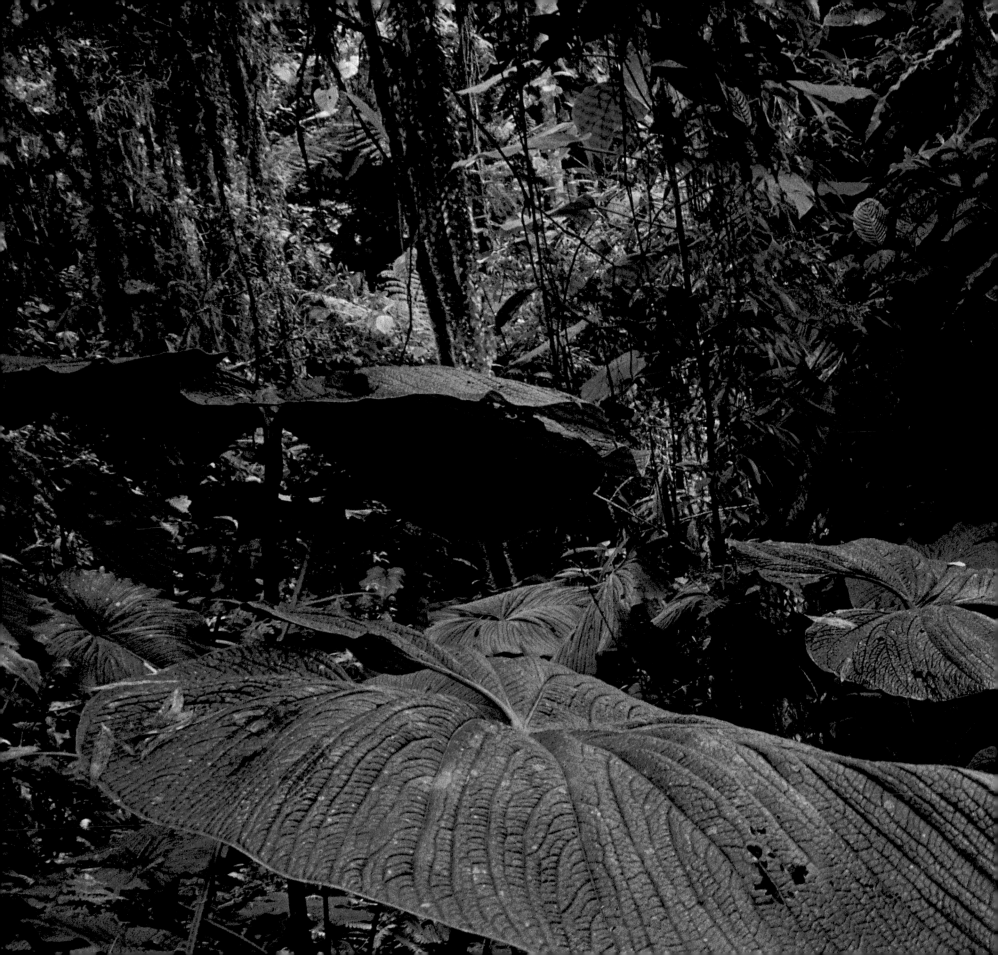

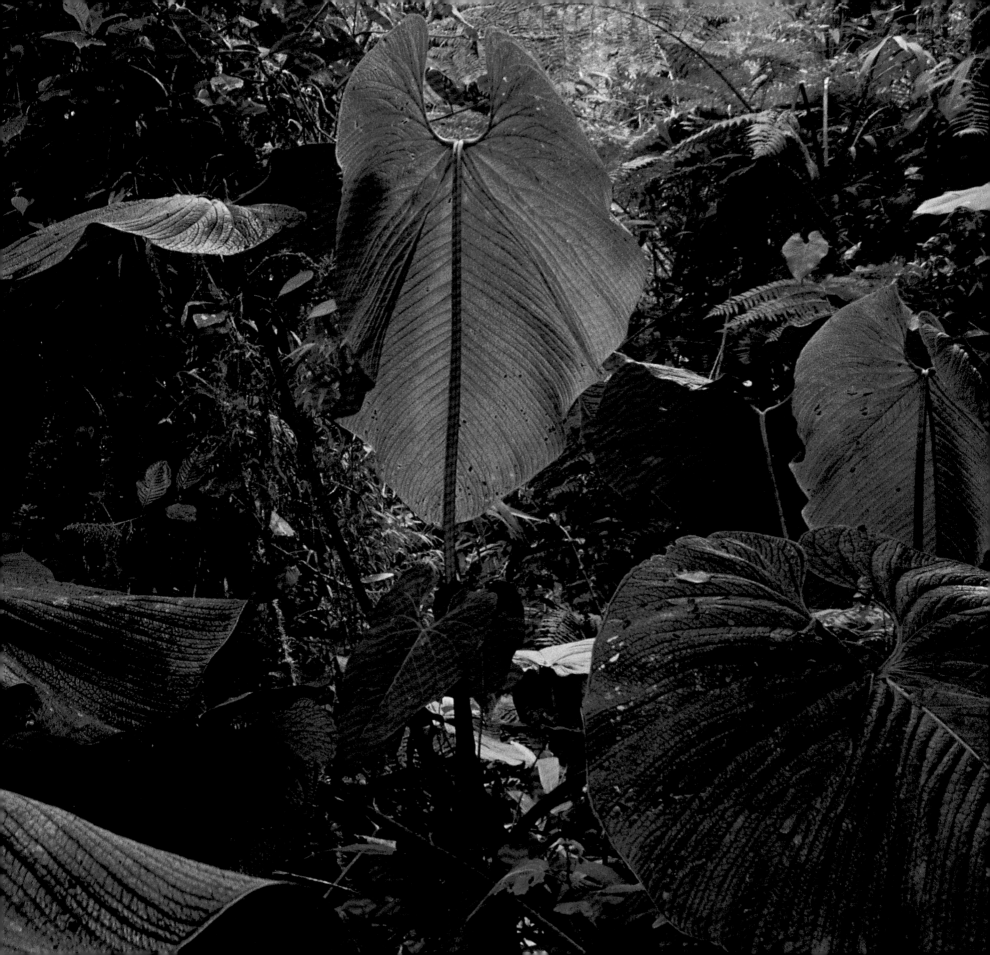

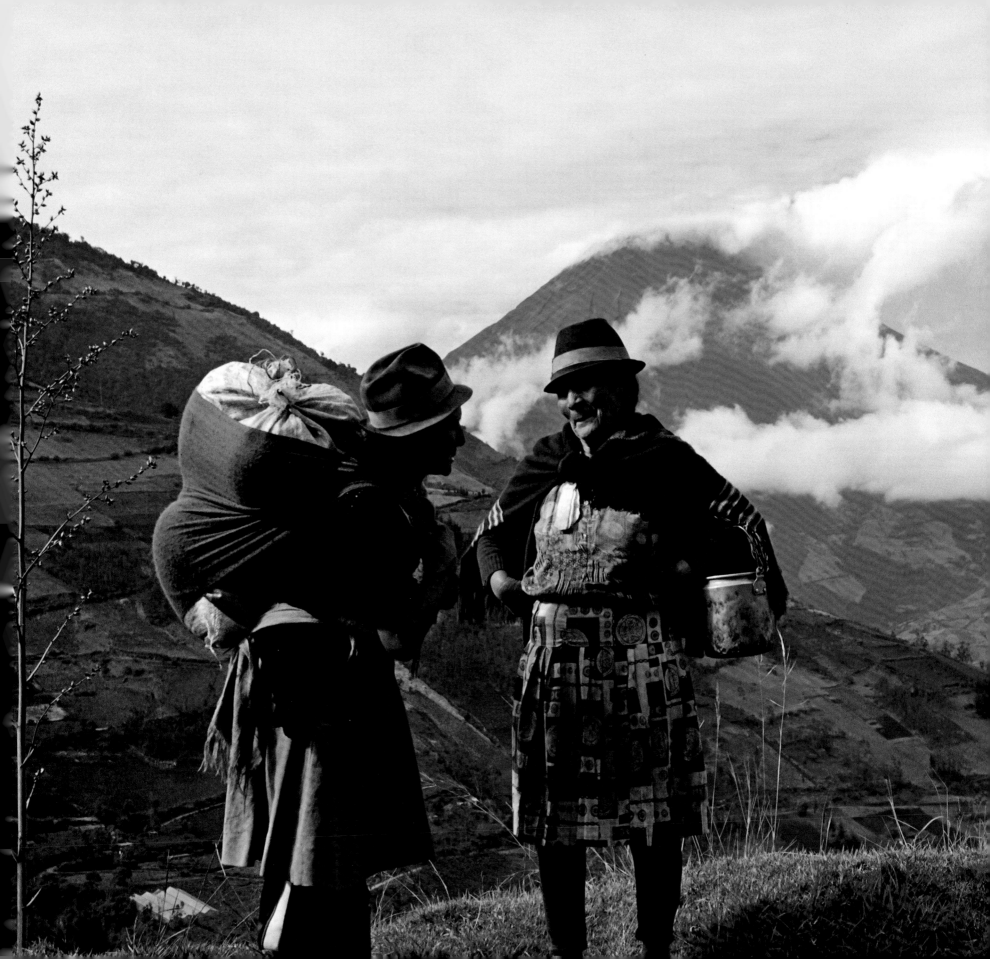

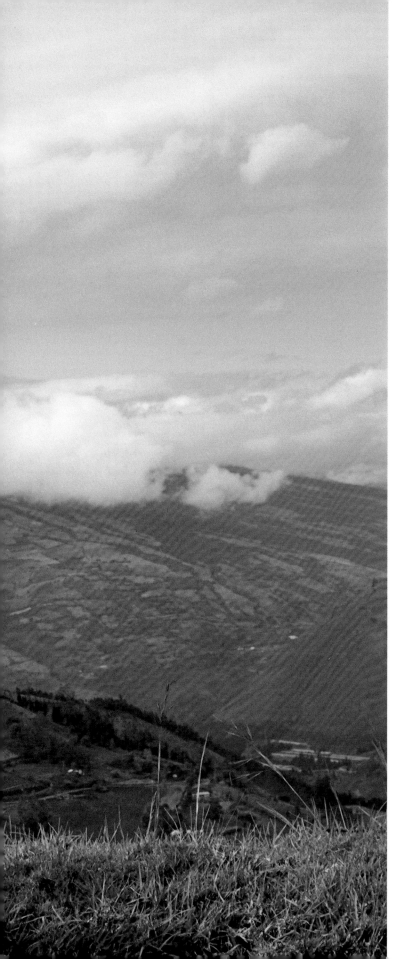

Survival is tenuous for hummingbird and human alike, for this is also the land of volcanoes. Fear of erupting volcanoes doesn't appear to touch the native folk. In this lush forest in the sky, 7,000 feet above sea, the local people live well past one hundred. Indian women farm the treacherously steep hillsides, which make it difficult for the flatlander to even stand upright. Native crops are grown that later fill head-balanced baskets these same women bring to the market. Generations of shared labor are in their hands, thick and wrinkled with layers of soil pressed into skin. Remnants of garments once intact swaddle their soft bodies in colorful bands of pattern and cloth. Their lives assume a natural rhythm. Eyes glitter as we pass; smiles formed by crooked teeth express what language lacks.

My disease becomes less relevant, disappearing in the clouds. In a place of constant beauty, good-humored crop tenders and a woman with fragile health blend together on steep mountainsides. There is something in this harsh yet abundant landscape that makes me fit in, something in this enduring place that makes me more accepting of my own body. Although I didn't come with an awareness of generations before being part of the land, now I feel it—healing is attunement and acceptance.

–Karen

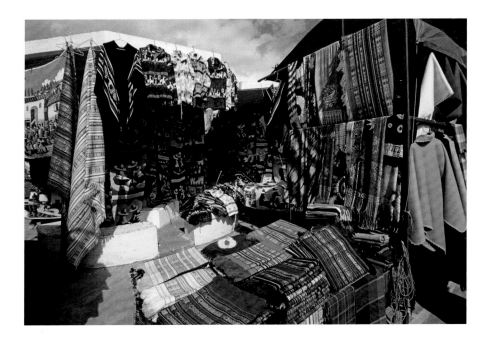

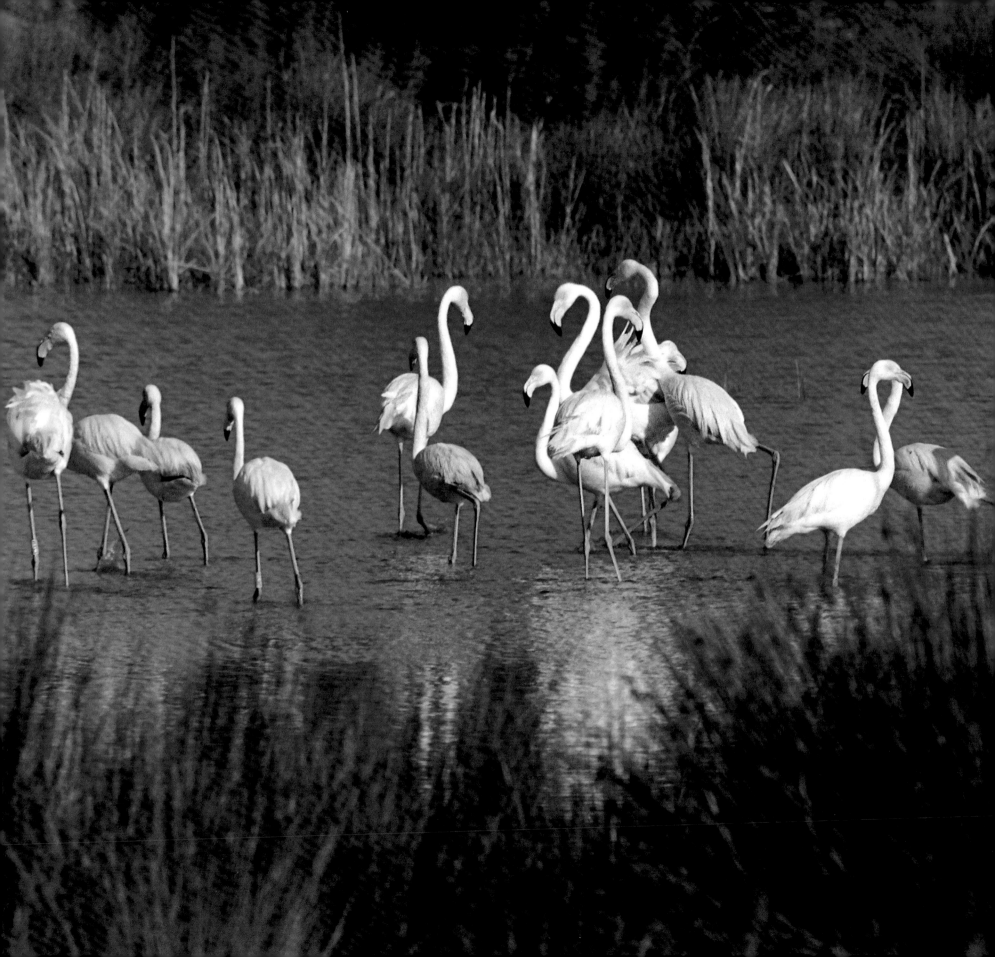

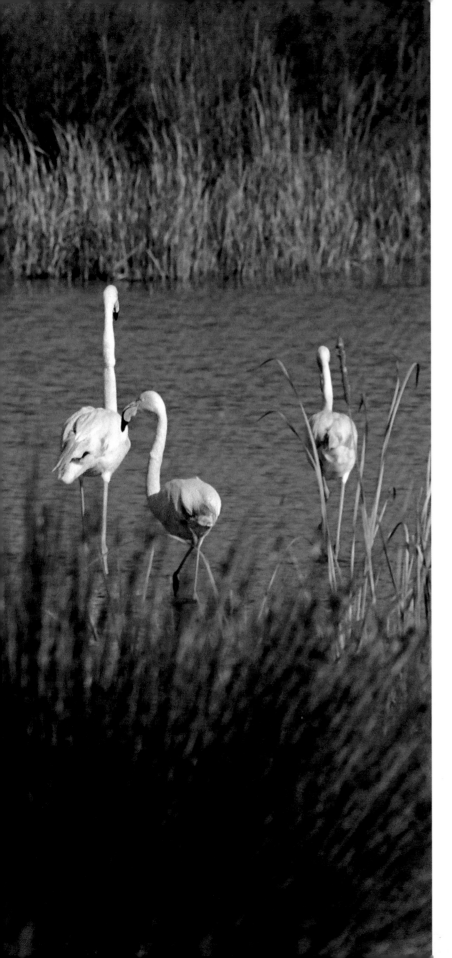

Black Bulls, White Horses
France

The Camargue is a marvel of human and natural engineering. This delta between the Mediterranean Sea and the Rhône River has been a center of religious and agricultural pursuits since the time of the Romans. It does not seem to have been touched by time, as if the ancient French culture remains. The natural sequence of tides, of salt remaining as tides withdrew, beckoned not only farming interests but the salt industry as well. The maintenance of the delta then required ambitious dikes and systems of monitored flows.

Wildlife, including abundant birds, has been preserved in the magnificent Parc Ornithologique. At first, I saw only the water mirroring the sky, a dusty, murky brown. Our existence was solitary in this landscape of unmoving water atop fields of young rice barely breaking the surface. There was almost no discerning above from below. It took time and attention to start seeing, like a meditation on not seeking, until the birds appeared.

The glorious pink flamingos, dancing for each other in a mating ritual we'd never understand, held us spellbound. Cameras raised, we began our creative dance, hoping to capture their wing or their touching or simply their mass, as there were hundreds now. Tim said quietly, "Use your fastest lens now. Go wide open to capture them with their quick, fluttering moves." Teacher reminded student of the challenge of light and speed—now—as the group rose above the water; perhaps I missed the lesson, but the glorious image I'll never forget.

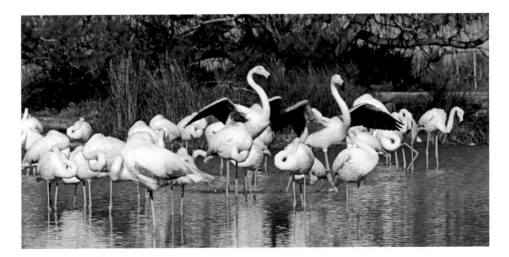

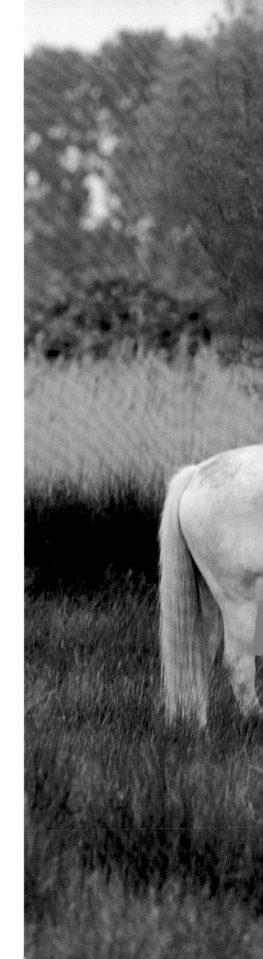

Birds weren't the only attraction in this corner of Provence. Black bulls and the white horses of Carmargue provided further glimpses of the ancient culture here. They were brought together in a tapestry of youth and bullfight for weekend entertainment. The "bullfight" we watched would best be described as acrobatic games of tease and run—no, vault—as the young men threw themselves over the wall to escape. The fun of that Sunday for locals was picnicking, while the horses and bulls of Camargue did what they've always done.

I reflected on feeling part of something more, part of the natural play of life. Granted, I don't think of life as "play," but I felt the powerful ebb and flow of the tides. A balancing force carried me, cared for me. That same force was healing me, lifting my body from the irregular "bio machine" of before, replacing it with new cells, new nerve fibers. Imagine, all the cells in our skeletons are replaced every seven years!

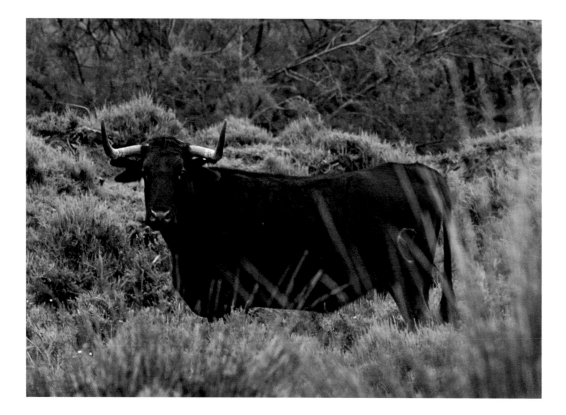

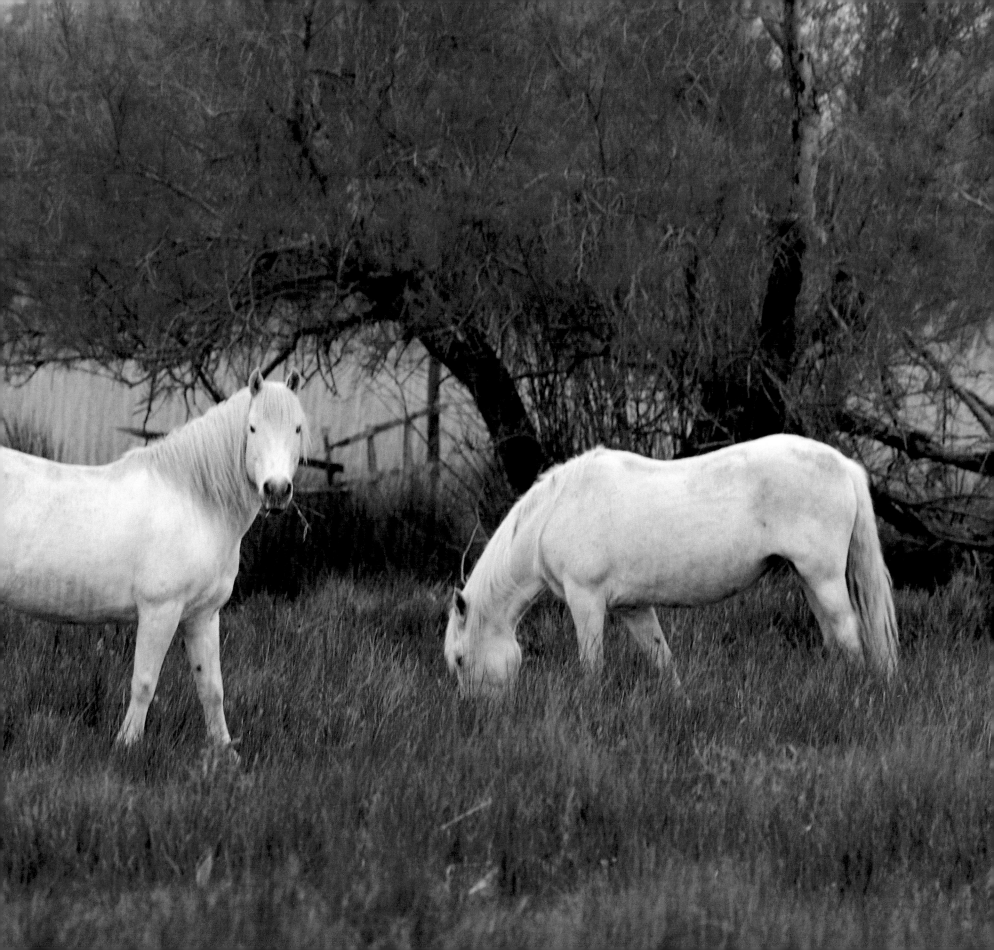

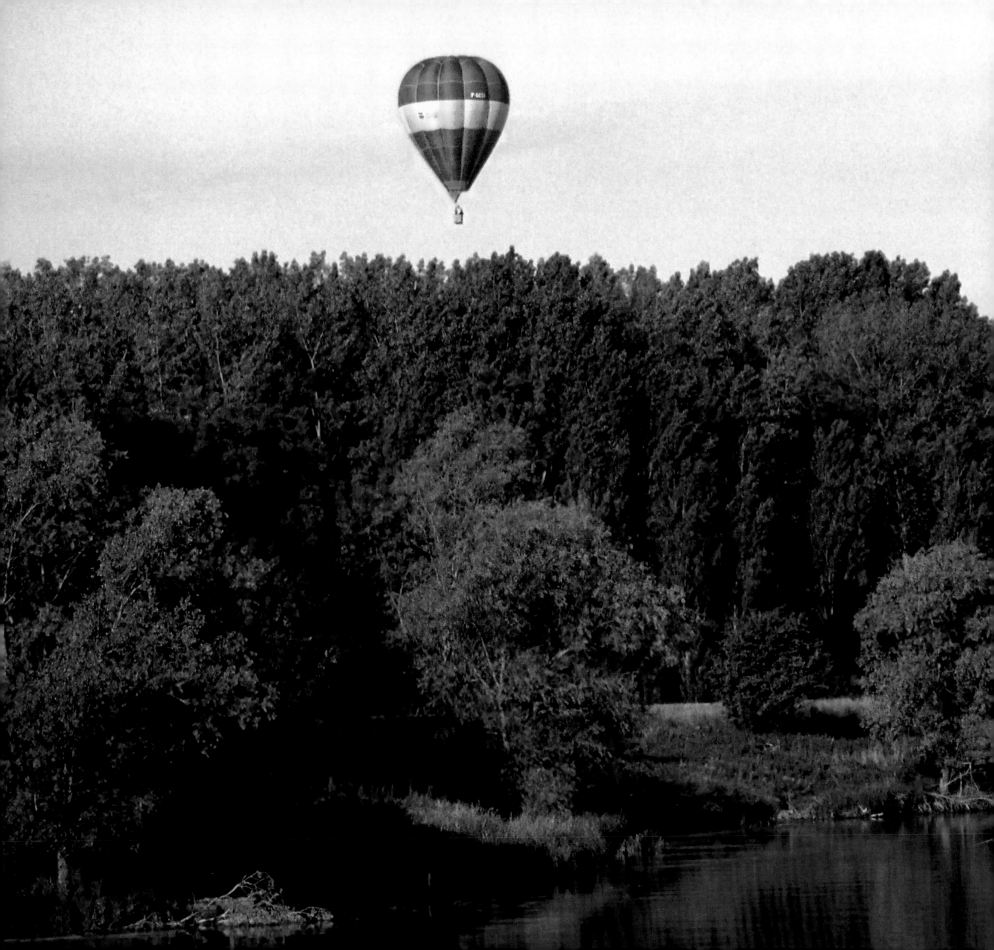

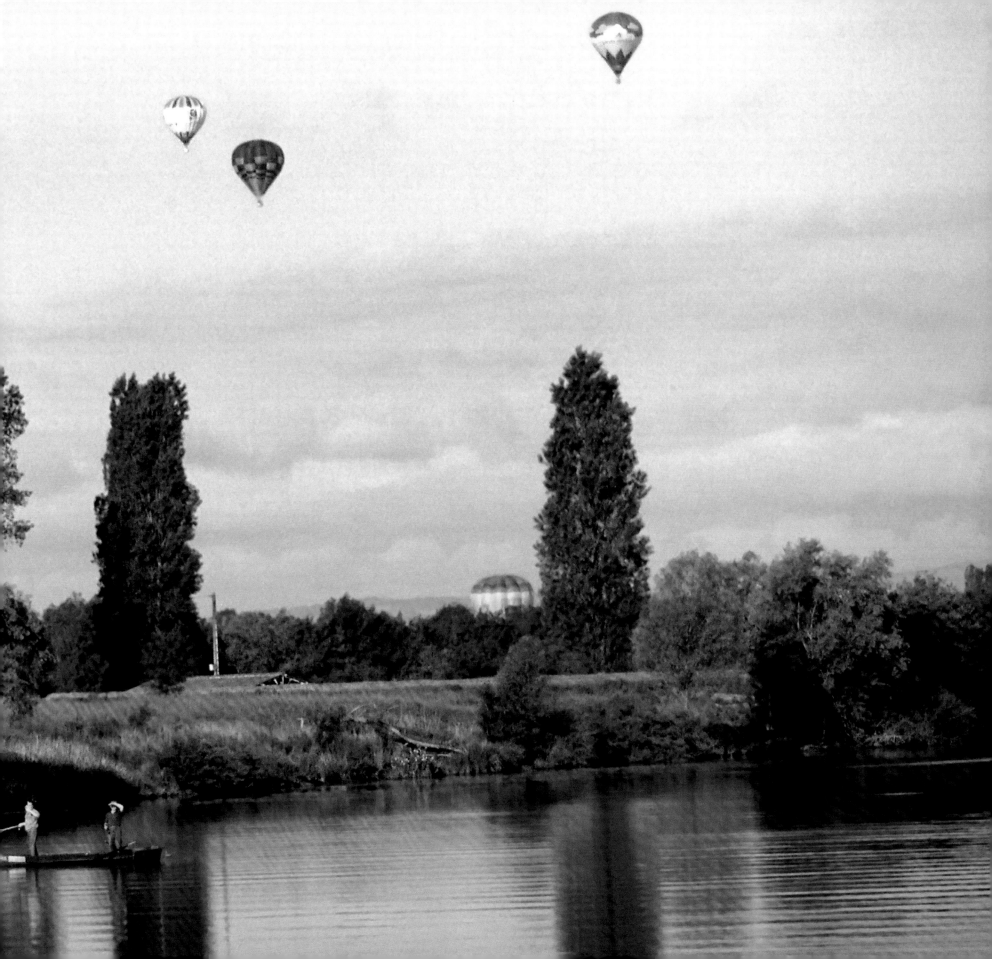

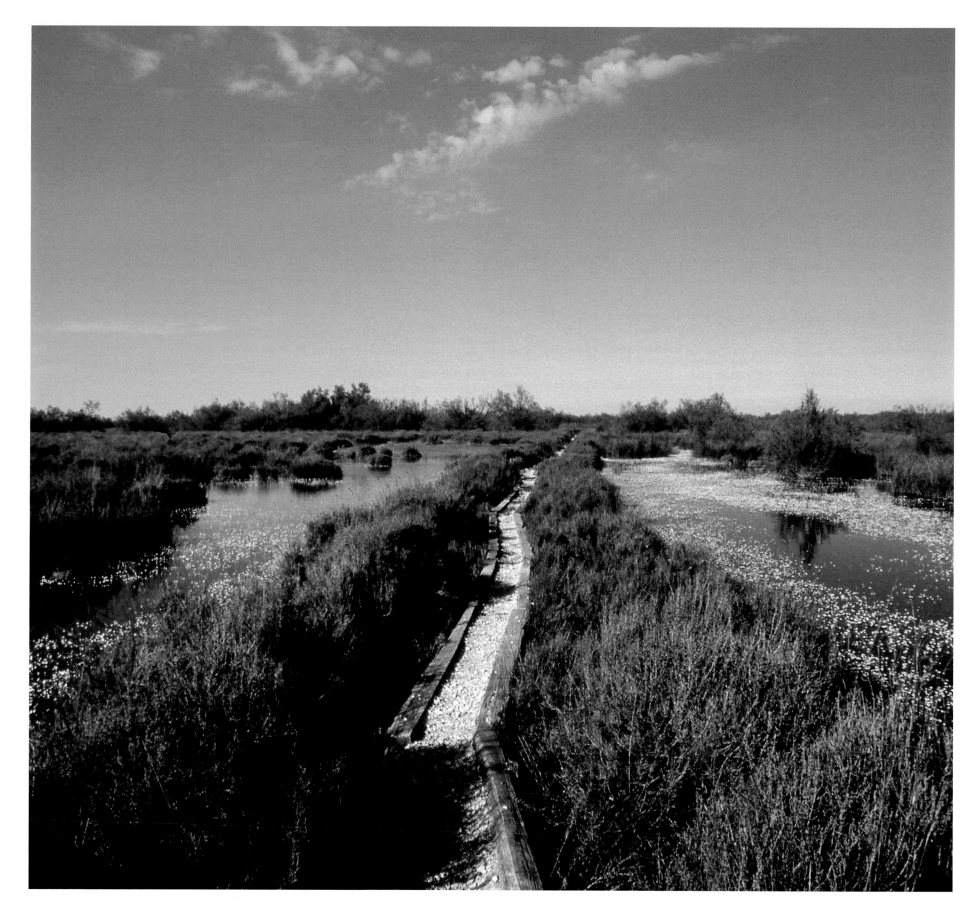

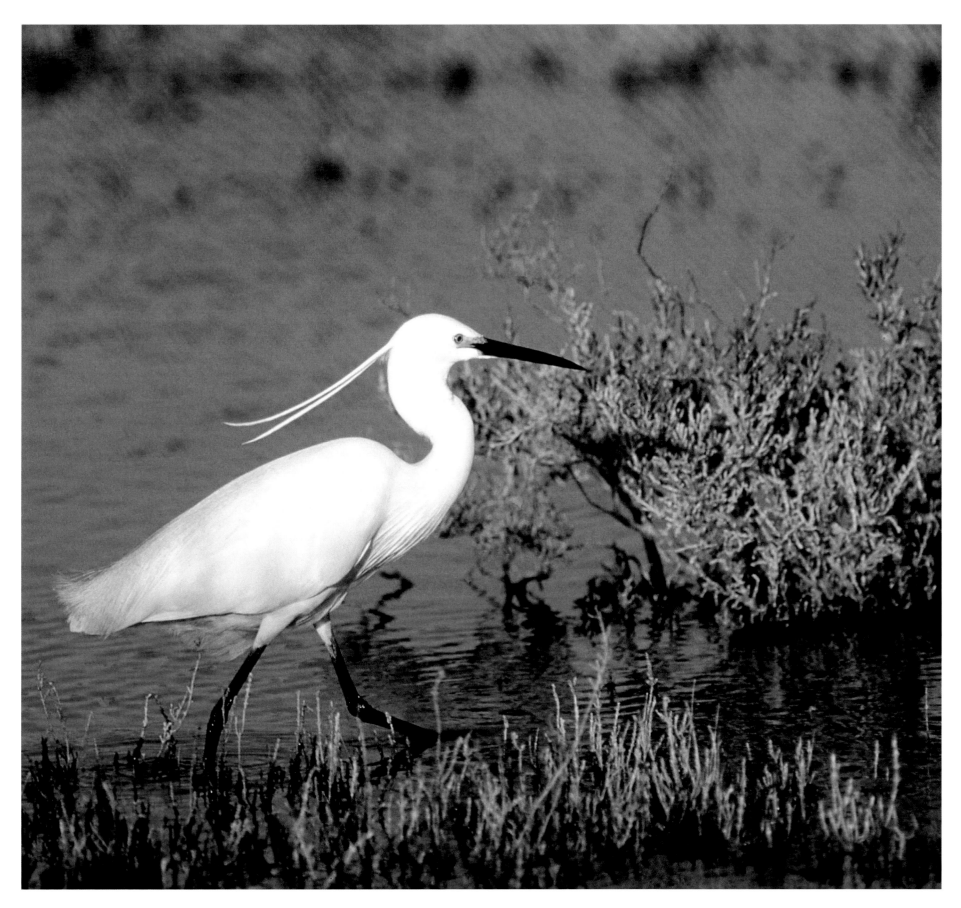

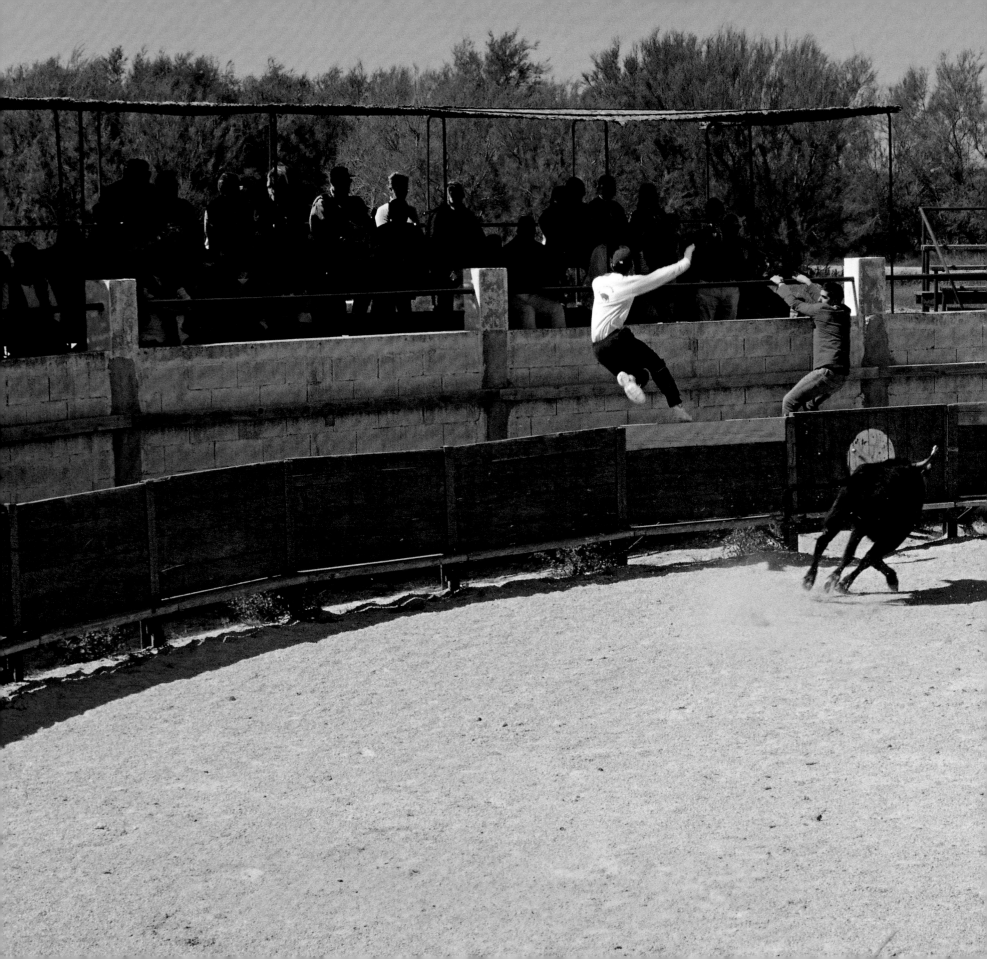

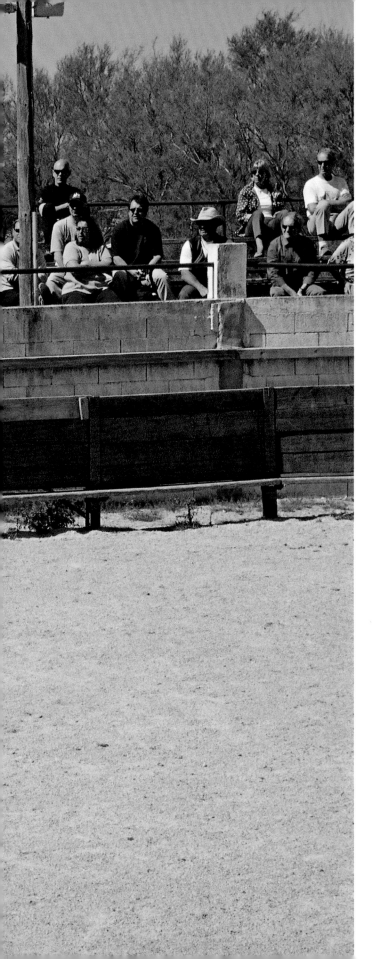

Having watched the kids hurl themselves over the wall, away from the bull, I realized how little I thought of my own back, now often a bit slouched. I needed to rediscover my natural posture, and regain the alignment that was lost somewhere behind desks and steering wheels or the defeat of MS. Finding a new uprightness, in vertebrae and in outlook, would be my gift from the Camargue.

While our trip was only to visit the Parc, when we learned of a balloon contest not far, we attended. Our spirits soared not only with the birds but with the glorious balloons, so smoothly lifting into the sky. My usual downward gaze was directed upward again. Retraining a body's stature usually takes more than a week, but our days in Provence brought me a lightness, an upward focus that was new. Being lifted away from the land, being elevated for a moment, reduced the drag of human embodiment. I barely remembered the years of not knowing whether I'd ever walk on trails or travel abroad. I knew the reality of a body that didn't respond when asked, as asked. This lightness enabled me to ignore the possibility that my body might again go awry. We were in the land of history and tradition, where life didn't seem to change, and maybe MS wouldn't take over. Or maybe it didn't matter.

I accepted that I wouldn't vault over the fence like the bull players, wouldn't go airborne in balloons, and that maybe health is a matter of perception, like finally seeing the birds in the mist. I would, as long as I was alive, be able to sense life around me. Participating in life might mean taking photos or writing or maybe just watching. I believed now in the forces of healing, imperceptible, like the tides.

–Karen

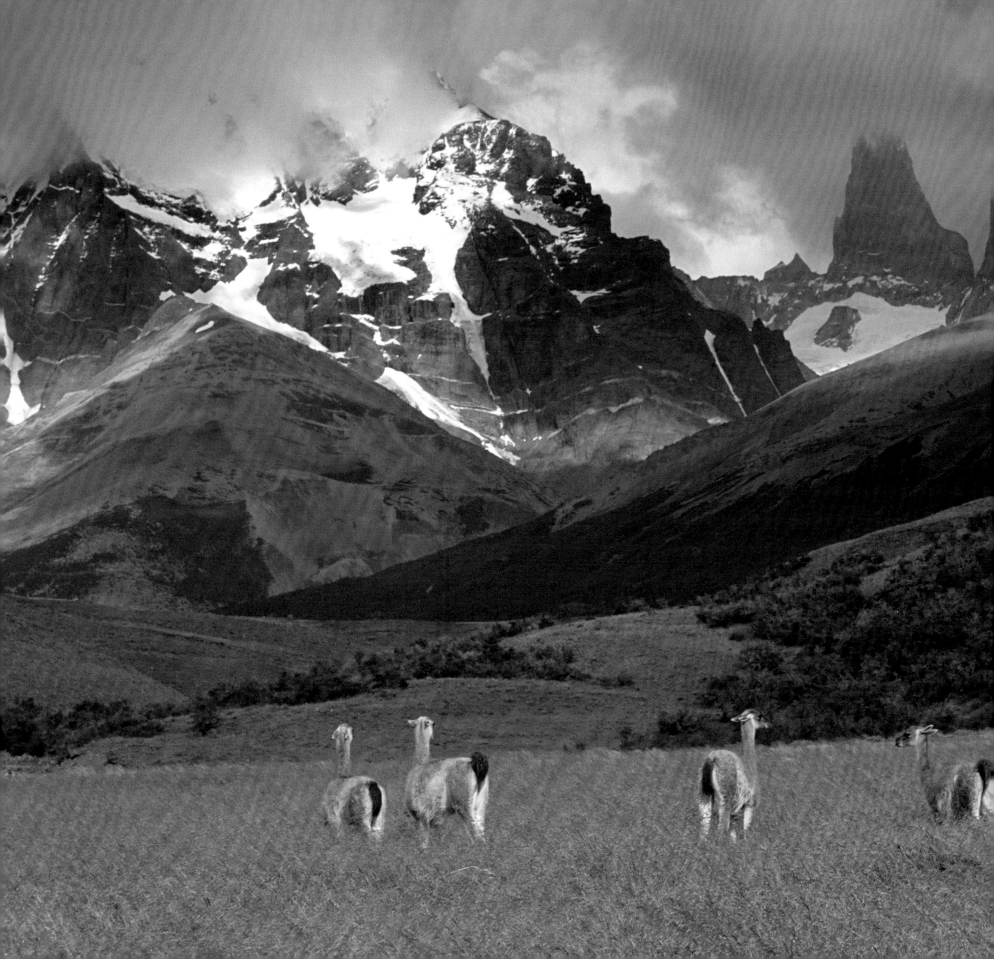

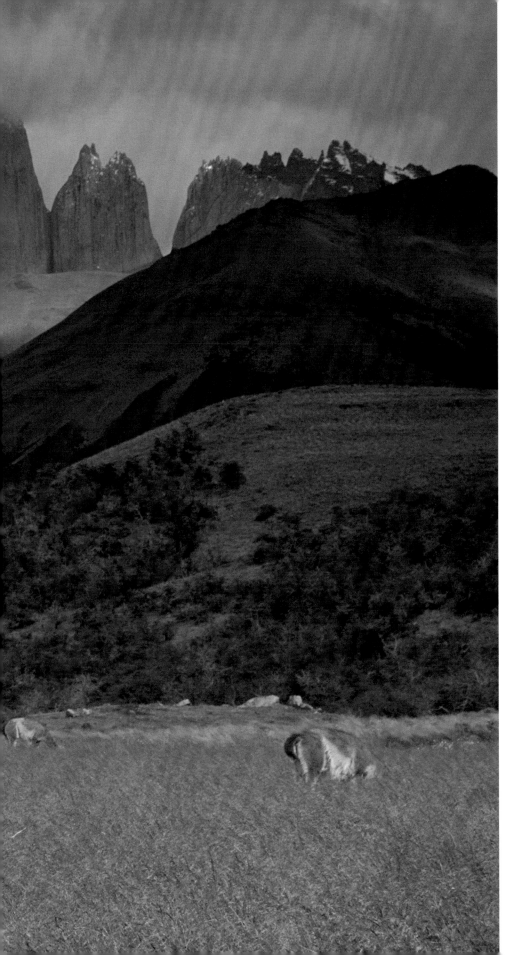

Birdsong and Silence
Chile

Mysterious, shrouded in blue clouds, Torres del Paine made a strong statement in this underbelly of America. This trip had started as a photography jaunt that allowed me to tag along with Tim and learn from a real pro. But I soon realized that merely capturing an image was a superficial adventure—nothing compared to my intimate encounter with nature and finding my true self on the back of a horse. My life in sickness had removed many choices, but now I had discovered that same condition could open a new depth of experience, a new capacity for awe. Maybe I was developing neural pathways as I rode, maybe not. But I was simply happier being with my horse. What an awesome lesson learned atop a mountain in Chile!

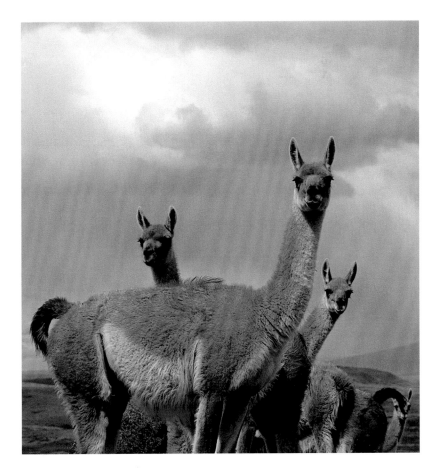

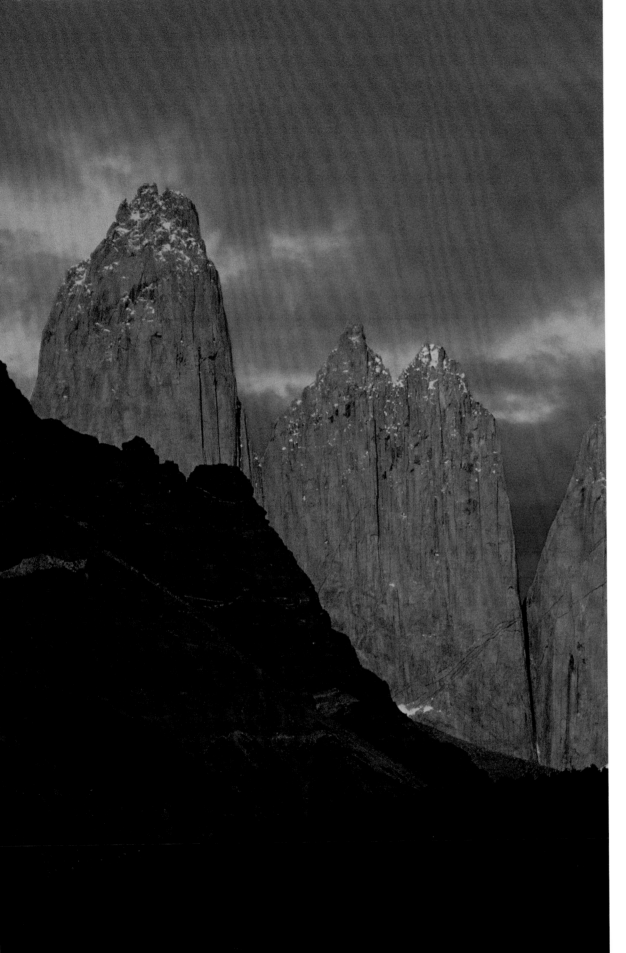

The magnificent jagged peaks of Torres del Paine are at the southernmost tip of the forlorn, unpopulated Americas. The wind blows fiercely here—even the birds are tossed about—and yet one morning we watched as a troop of intrepid international trekkers appeared with backpacks and walking sticks. They spoke various languages, were young and old, and had an apparent bottomless reservoir of excitement. We wondered how their nights would find them as the trail would not be easy. Not only a hostile wind with rain, but also mud, and a difficult path of ascents and descents, lay ahead on a five-day or seven-day circuit of the major mountain of Torres del Paine, the Massif. Some of them would be able to stay in a refugio for the night, but only those who had planned ahead and prepaid.

Earlier in my life, I had spent summers working in national parks in California and Montana so that I could spend every free moment hefting a backpack and hiking in the mountains. That was prior to midlife neurological and physical change, prior to the loss of balance, heavy legs, arms that didn't respond—all the various symptoms that came as a surprise and then left. While preparing for my trip to Torres del Paine, I could have trained hard and then chosen a slower, longer way up so that I could have been part of this group activity. But I didn't want to be dependent on others, perhaps hampering their already challenging path.

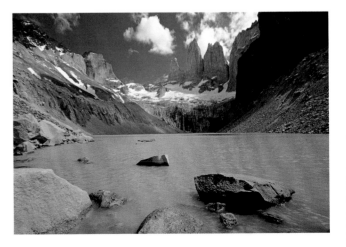

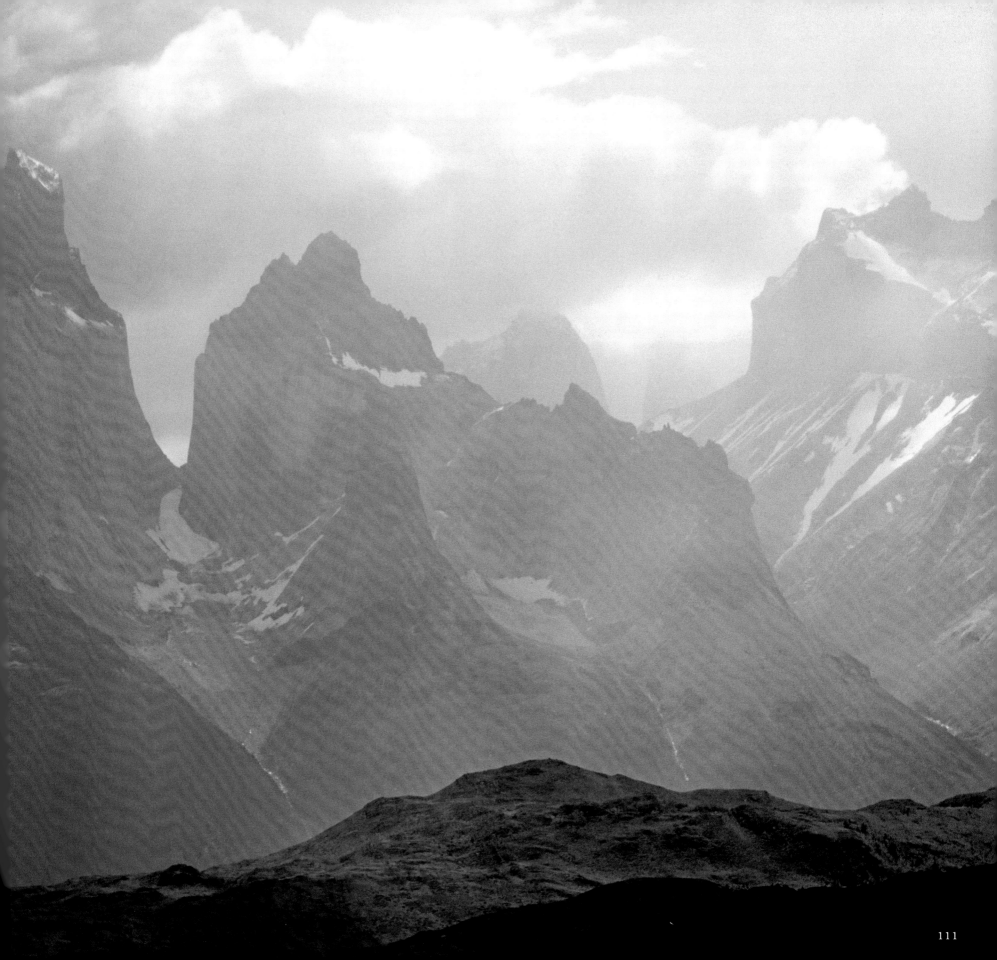

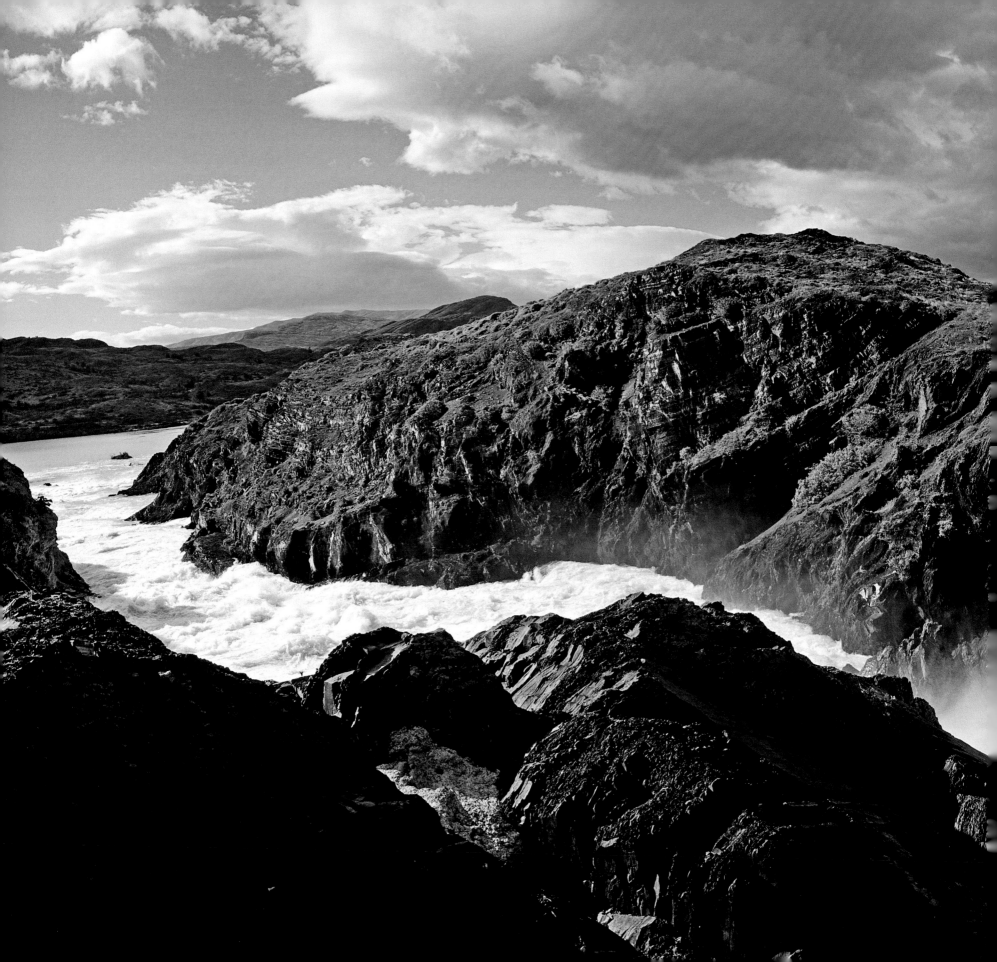

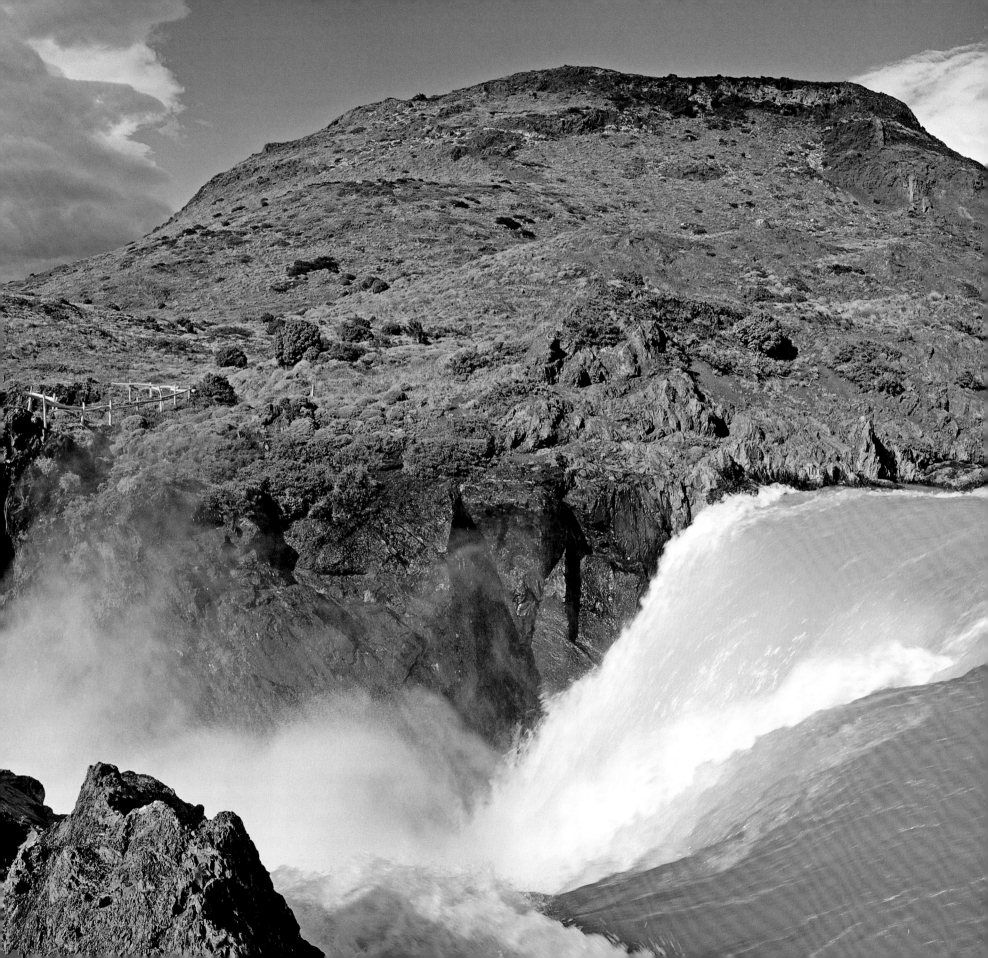

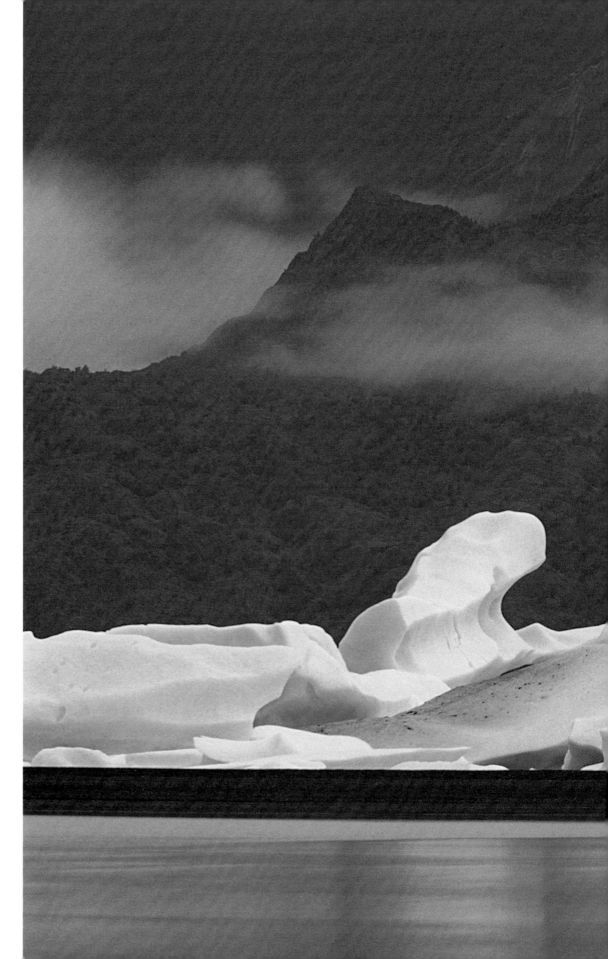

I didn't want to be tromping along in the mud for days anyway, because I knew from experience with this confounding condition that if I let myself wallow in something like self-pity, I would pay, very likely have an "episode." I could wake up partially paralyzed, with legs that didn't listen or a hand that couldn't grasp. Being in this incredible, wild beauty demanded I participate in some way beyond taking photographs. I wanted to be like my puppy, his first time at the beach, crazed by the smells of the sea, the water rushing at him in waves, afraid to rush back at those waves and settling for obsessive rolling in the stinky seaweed. How could I roll in this experience of Torres del Paine?

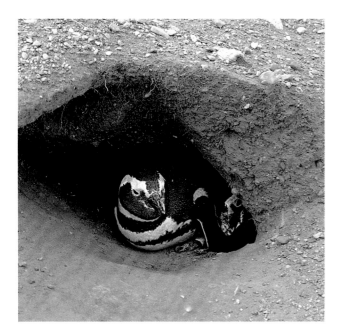

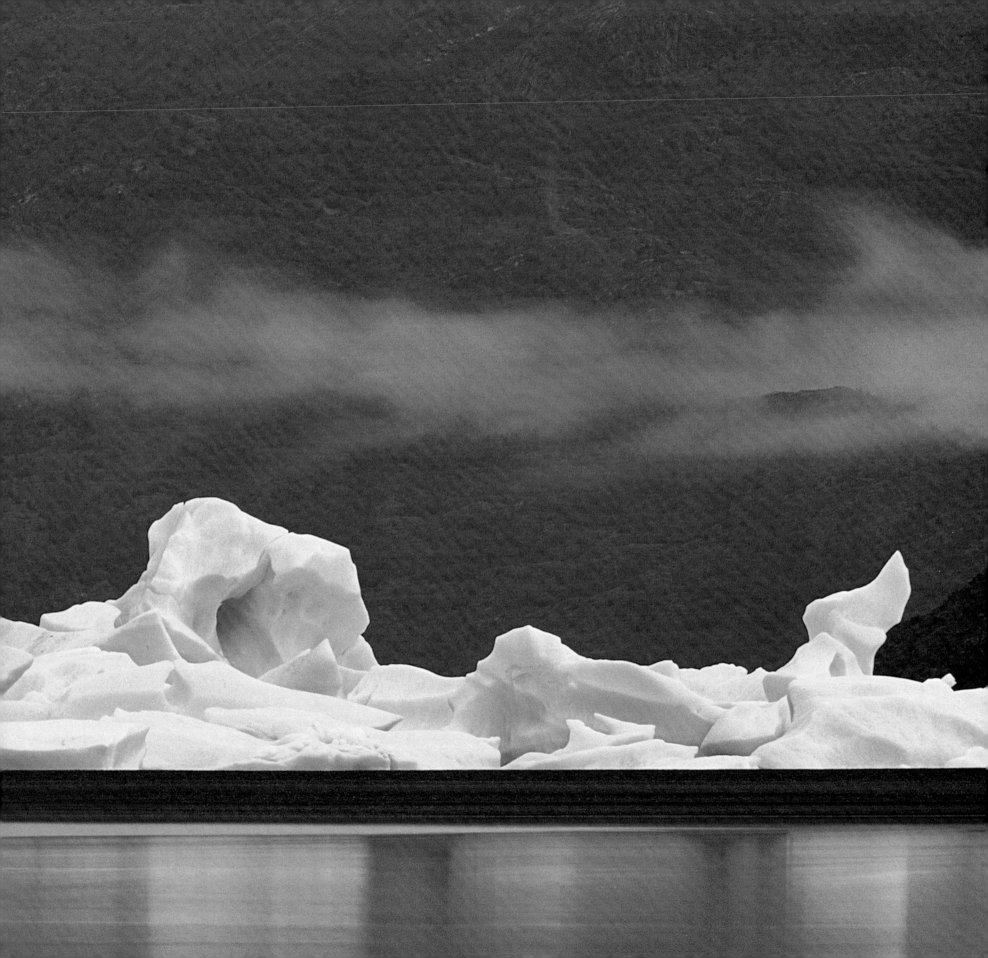

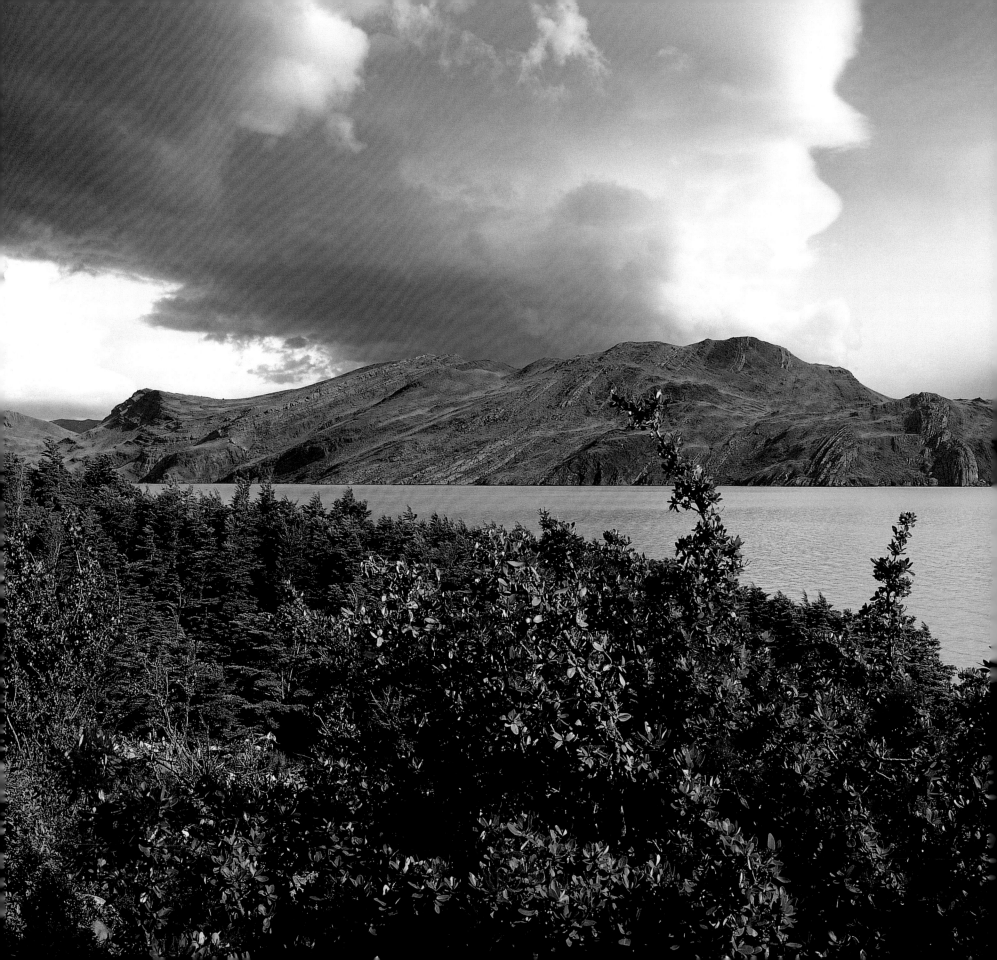

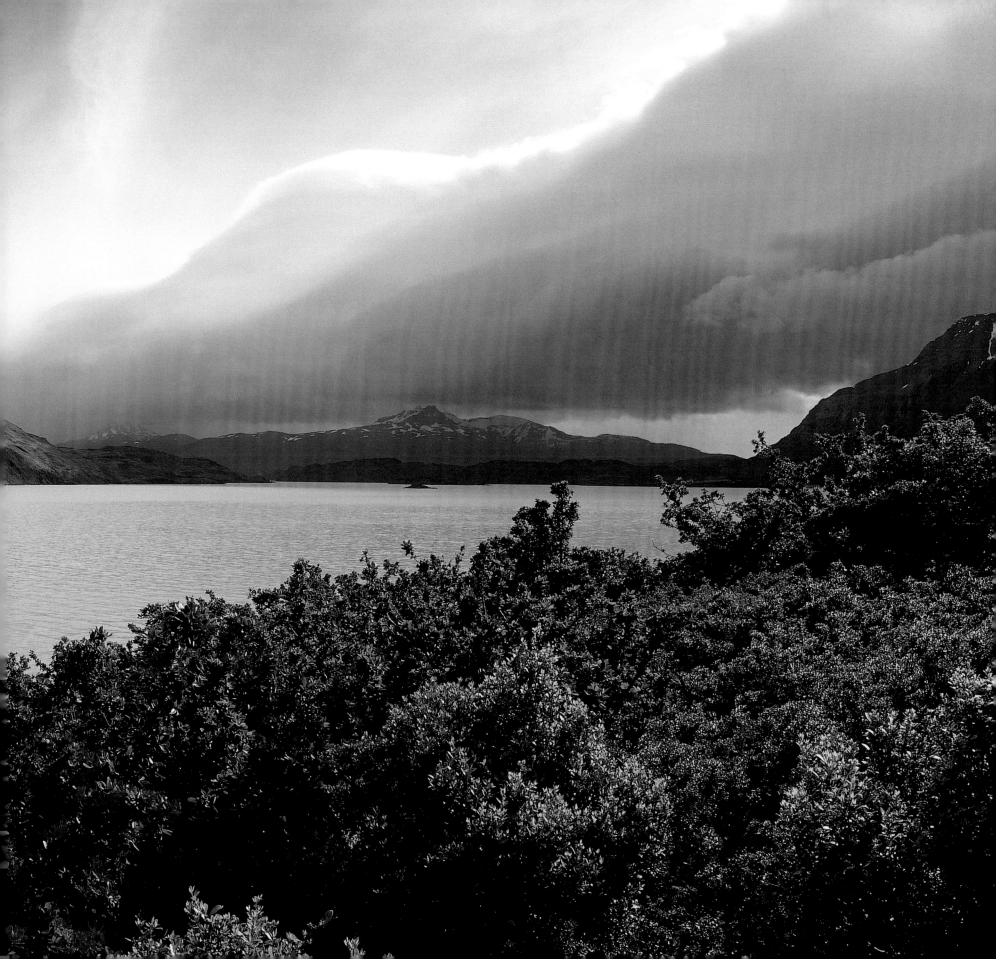

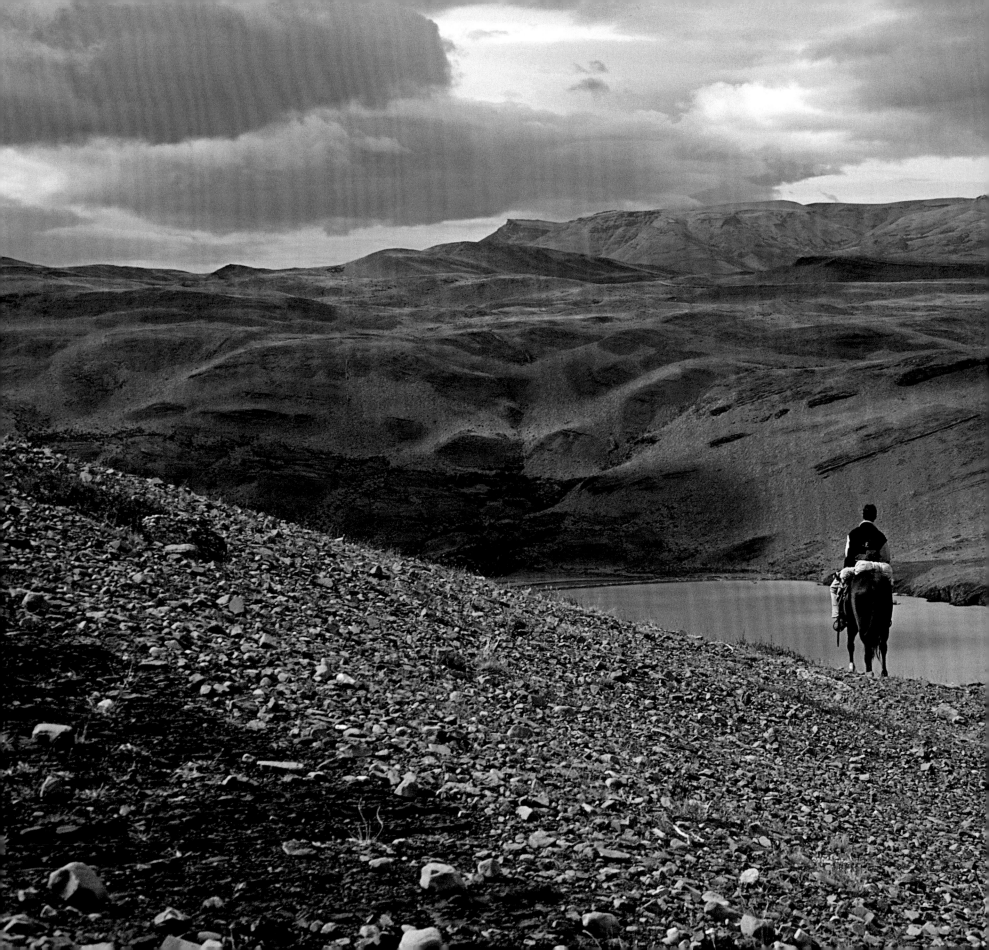

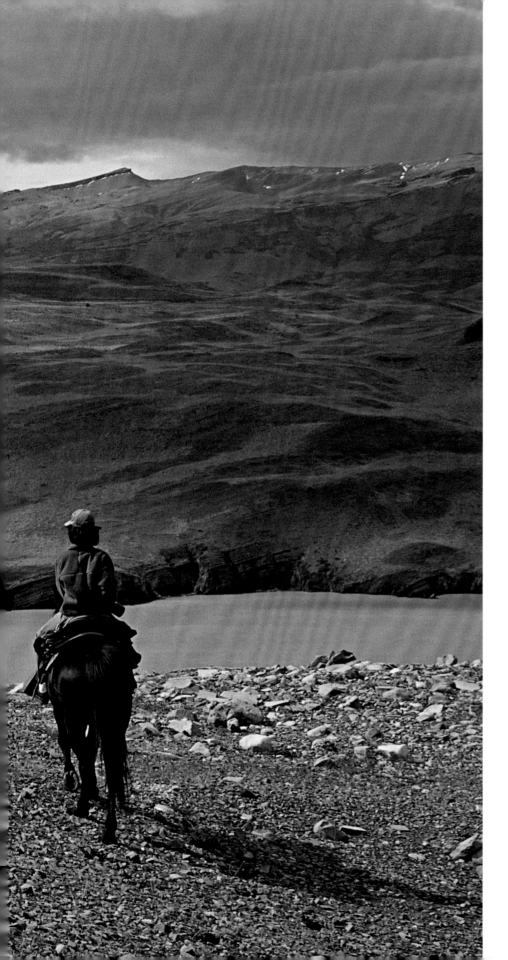

The next day my question was answered: Get on a Chilean pony and ride! We were guided by a gaucho who spoke little English and clearly loved his land. We went into the mountains, crossed the plains high above, and encountered wild guanaco not startled by our appearance. We were spellbound by the beauty of a turquoise lake in the middle of a rocky landscape that was perfectly still in spite of the high winds. We were so alone there, as if humankind had never stepped upon this land before us. Even our gaucho guide seemed more a part of the landscape than an intruder. Our closeness with nature in those moments was pure and integrated; our presence and the clouds above were reflected in our azure lake. The silence was broken only by rare bird cries and constant wind, reminding us that even the eons of time could not alter this pristine place.

My disease hadn't stopped me. The perceived insurmountable challenge of my physical limitation was transformed when I began to enjoy daily horseback rides. Perhaps for reasons of concentration, body balance, and the symmetry of motion needed to successfully ride a horse, my symptoms of multiple sclerosis diminished. By being open to asking for more that afternoon in front of Torres del Paine Massif, I had been shown fabulous vistas and a new life with a horse. Debilitating diseases can steal away a person's belief in his or her right to live a full life. We may not realize to what extent we define ourselves by our limitations, even if they are temporary. Overcoming my sense of being bottled up reminded me of a frog experiment I once read about. The amphibian had incredible leg strength, and yet it would not attempt to leap out of an open jar, because, in a previous experiment, the jar had a lid. The poor frog was living in the past, just like many human beings who quit reaching.

To speak of healing as a separate act, such as a doctor treating a patient, would be so misunderstood in this environment. Only natural rhythms and energies prevailed. They carried me away from the mind-body paralysis I had been living with. By allowing a new story to replace the old one that refused to take me where I wanted to go, I discovered not only a different carrier—horse—but also a new me. As a horseback rider, I acquired new powers and merged into the landscape, becoming whole in this arid, ancient, wild place.

—Karen

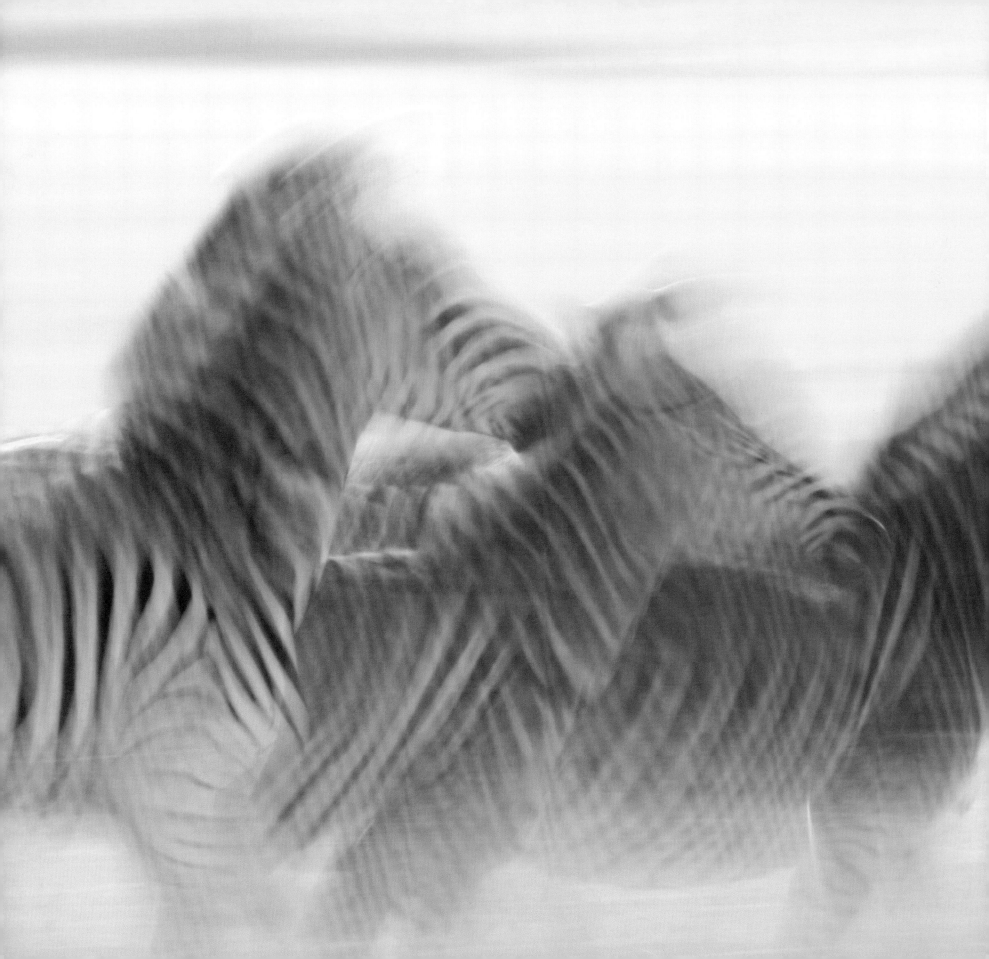

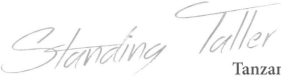

Home. It swept over me in the humid heat as we crossed the tarmac. Was there something in the air? Dust stirred by the tracks of our ancestors? It entered my body and awakened a collective memory, a powerful sense of returning. We poured into the customs room to complete our visas, sectioning off into lines that quickly tangled. I found myself staring at the ceiling fan, spreading its hot air in a chorus of creaks and groans. A large moth suddenly found me in the crowd. Shocked by its rapid approach, I held my breath. Wings tickled my neck, and away it flew. It would seem I had received a kiss from Africa.

In the Serengeti, diversity and coexistence are demonstrated in every interaction and encourage the visitor to surmise lessons for our own species. The migrations, linking animal with food source, reveal an interdependency that provides for all. While one animal may nibble the tip, the mid-layer of grass will be eaten by a different creature, which in turn allows others to receive nourishment. It is not just in feeding patterns that we see this integration. A zebra's keen memory and superior vision enable it to lead the migration; the wildebeest who follows assists by finding water. Together they find their way.

Watching the endless array of stripes, unique to each zebra, or the cheetah's tail balancing its speeding body, I marveled at form and movement. Wildebeest bucked across the plains in a stumbling yet flamboyant gait; an outline lifted from a Paleolithic cave painting had come out to play! A thin, pink line of distant flamingos shimmered like a mirage along the horizon. Under the acacia, sleeping lions sprawled, and birds sat on high branches like radiant jewels.

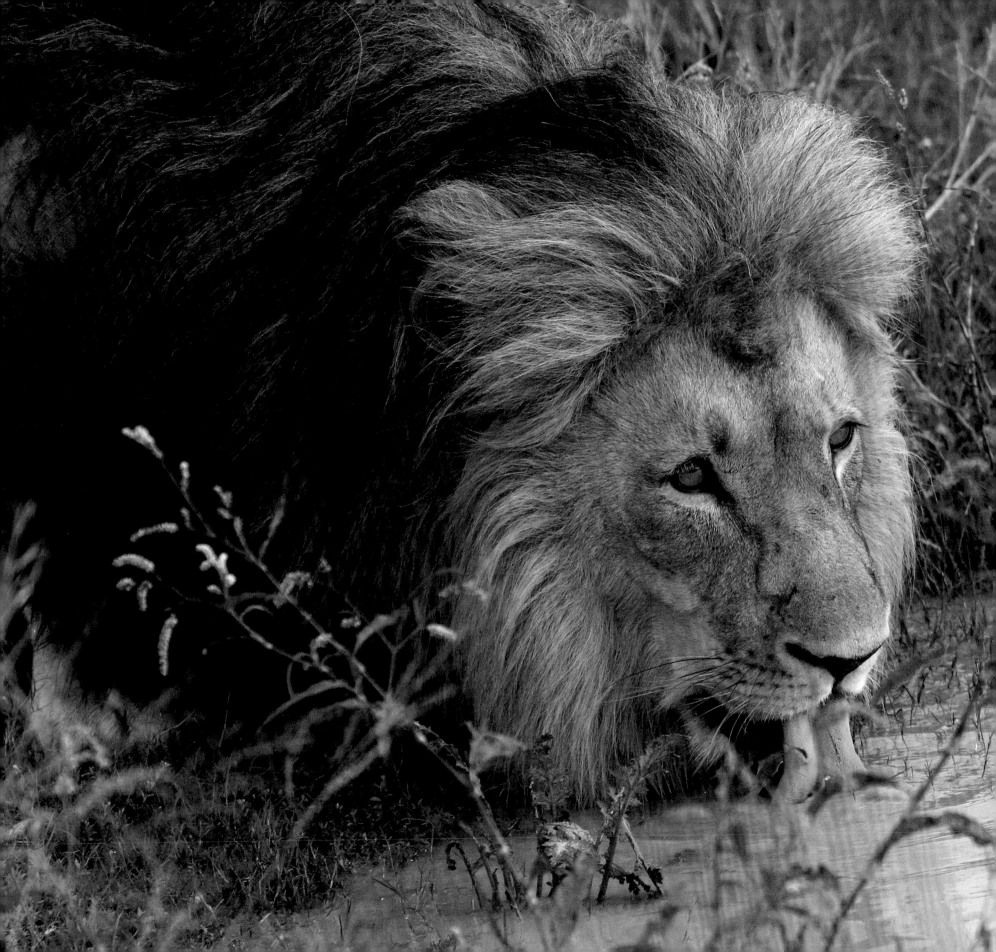

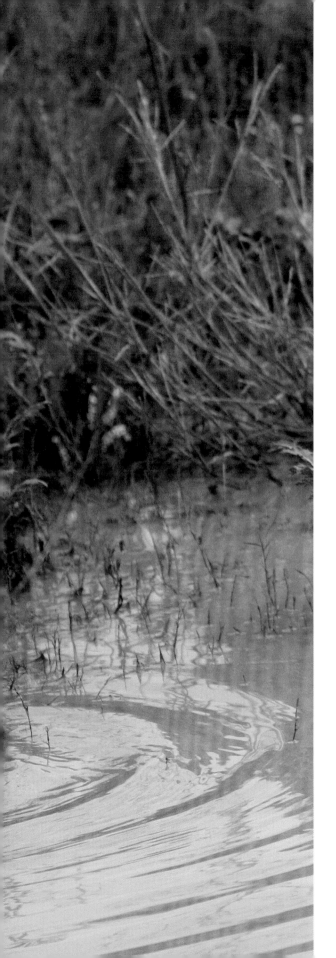

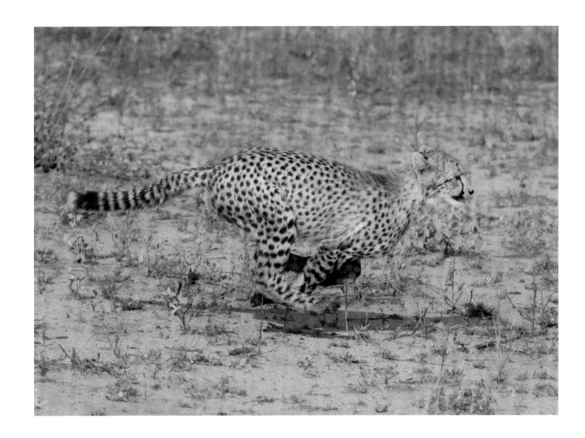

We stayed in a tent camp where restless animals passed in their nocturnal day. The noises of the hunt charged my body. An instinct to survive spoke louder than sleep. Lying alert in my cot, I let my ears roam the space my eyes could not see. Rapid exhalations sounded so close to the canvas wall that I felt as if I were being hunted. Do I know how to survive? I asked myself. What are my tools? I contemplated these self-preserving impulses in muscle and mind. As the sun rose, my gratitude for the return of light was accompanied by a wish to live in the fullness of every moment.

For the first two days of our eight-day trek to the rooftop of Africa, I followed in the footsteps of my guide. Unsteady in my own hiking boots, I received an entire education from his imprints. I studied how he shifted his weight, how he turned his feet on slippery descents or chose rocks along a river crossing. I gradually raised my head and began to find my own steps. His father had been bringing him to the mountain since he was twelve. At age seventeen, he was told he was ready to make the trek alone. The mountain had revealed many sides in these years of training and observation. I would safely climb Kilimanjaro because of a father who had taught a son who was now teaching me.

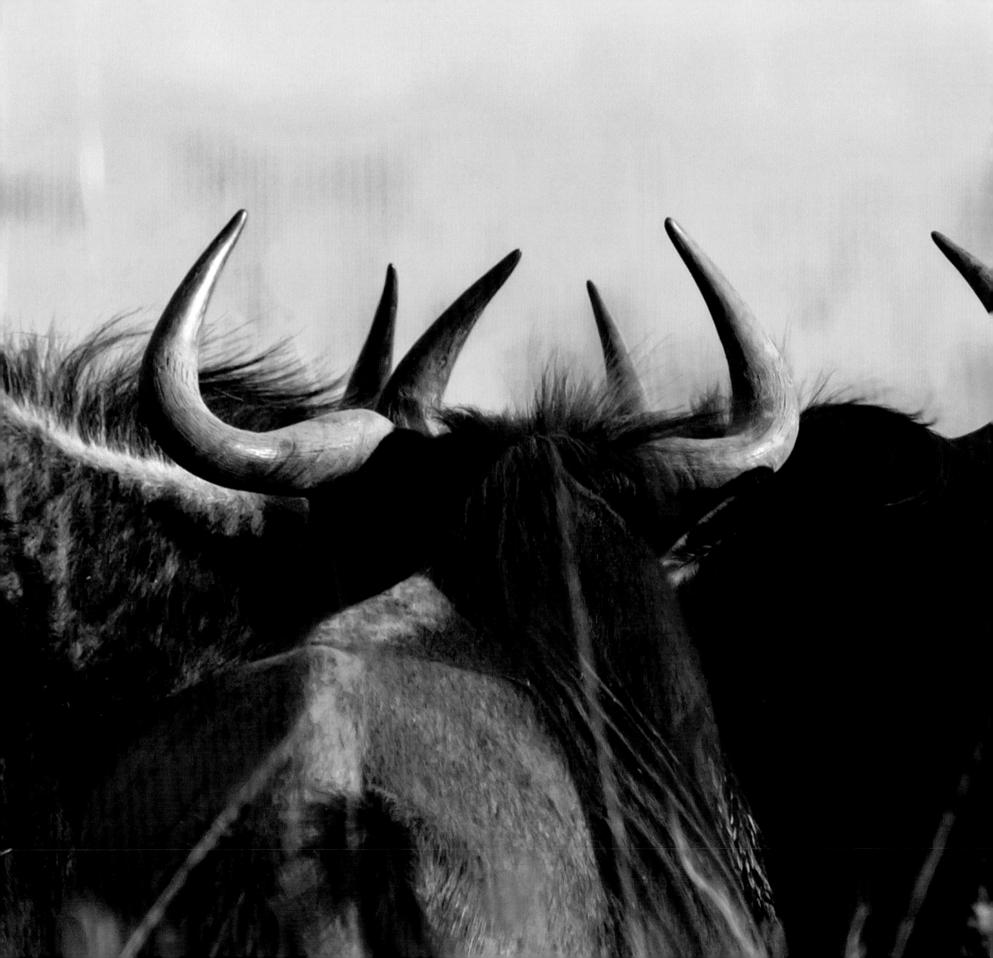

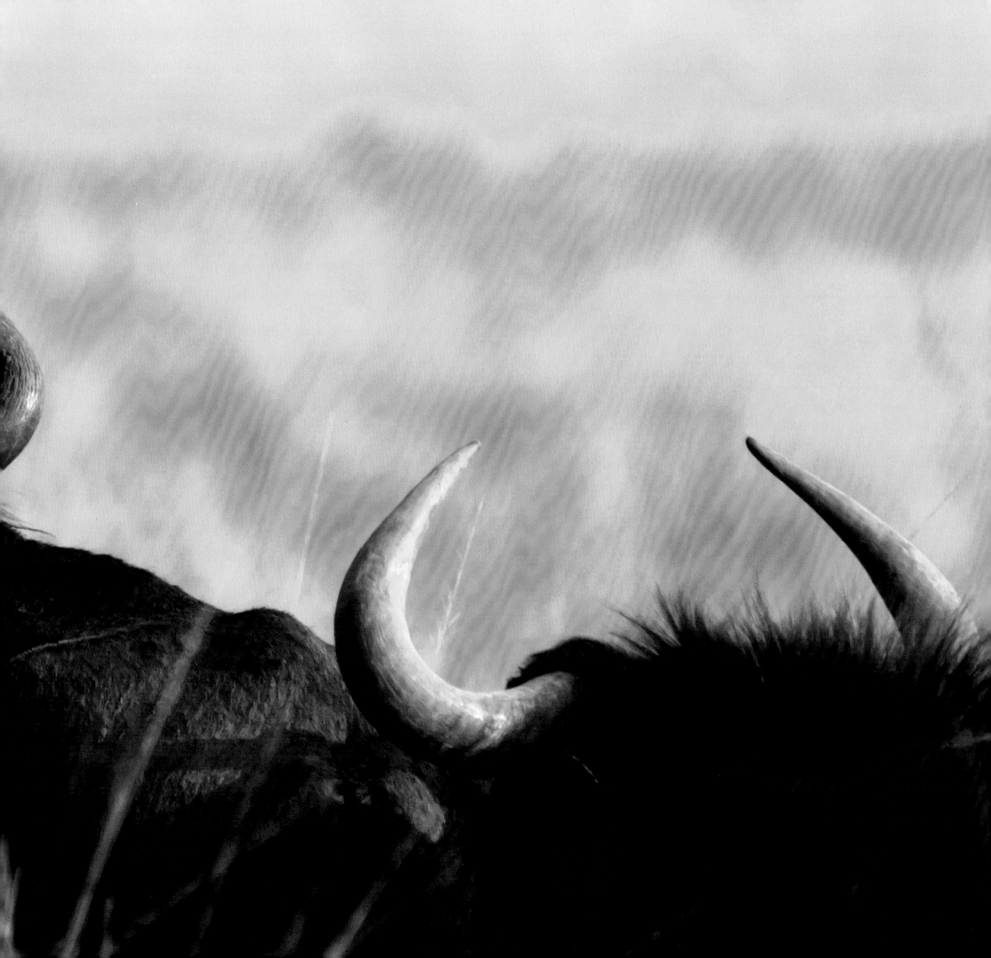

During the hike, I had been asked if I felt afraid. With snow blindness and altitude sickness forcing climbers and porters to descend prematurely, there were reasons for alarm. I found, however, my answer came immediately: I have no fear. To what would I attribute such fearlessness? This trip represented a journey into the unknown. With a mind-set unlimited by judgment, I held no expectations, and fear had no place to lodge itself.

There are many ways to reach the top, and all of them present challenges. For Mount Kilimanjaro, there are two approaches. One may walk a highway of sorts, rather wide and often covered in gravel. It bears little relation to the natural curves of the mountain—a miserable route that most climbers take up and down. Approaching from the other side, my companions and I made our own path to the summit. Our summit required ice axes. For minutes at a time, we waited and watched our guide as he tested where our course would turn. At times, deep snow pulled at us like quicksand. It was on this path that my body touched the bones of the mountain.

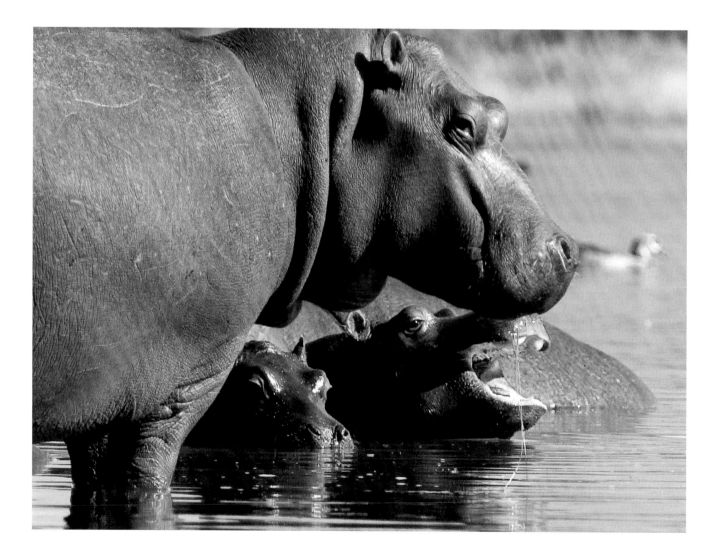

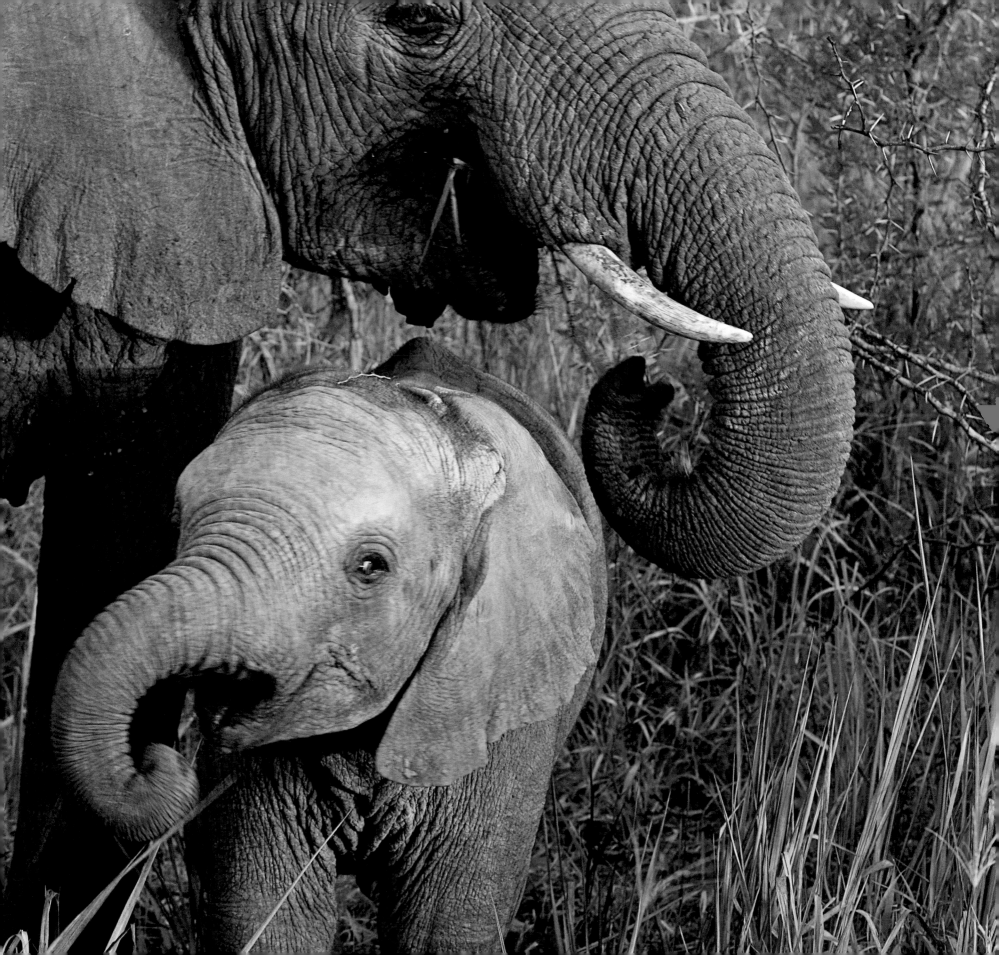

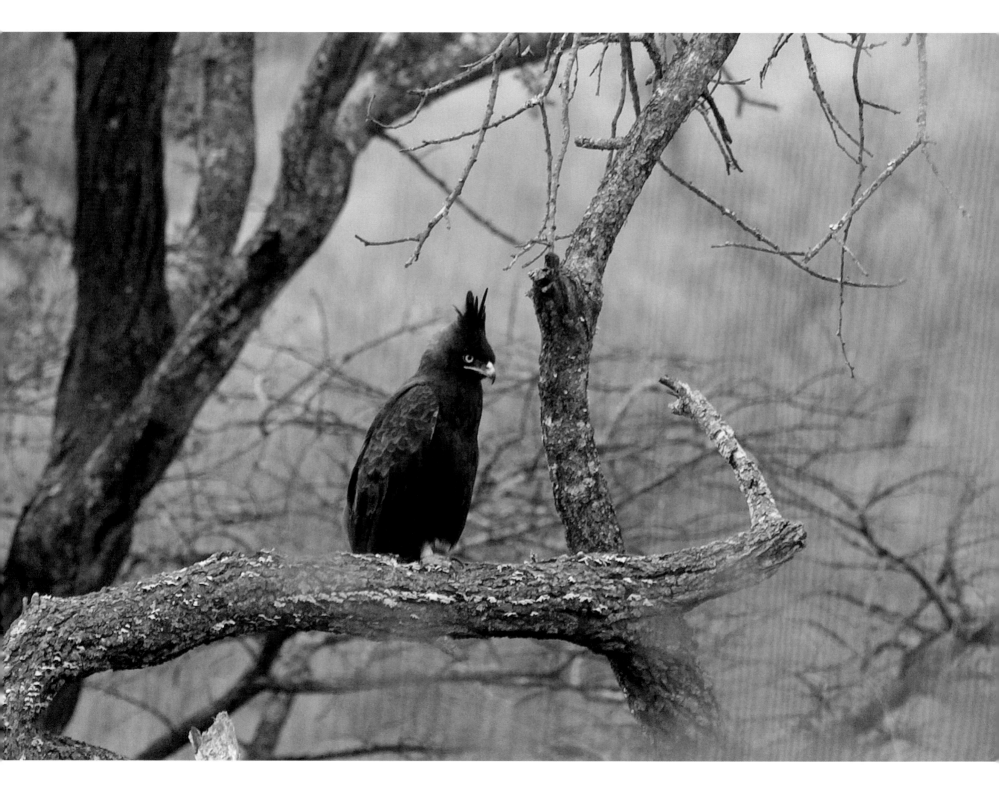

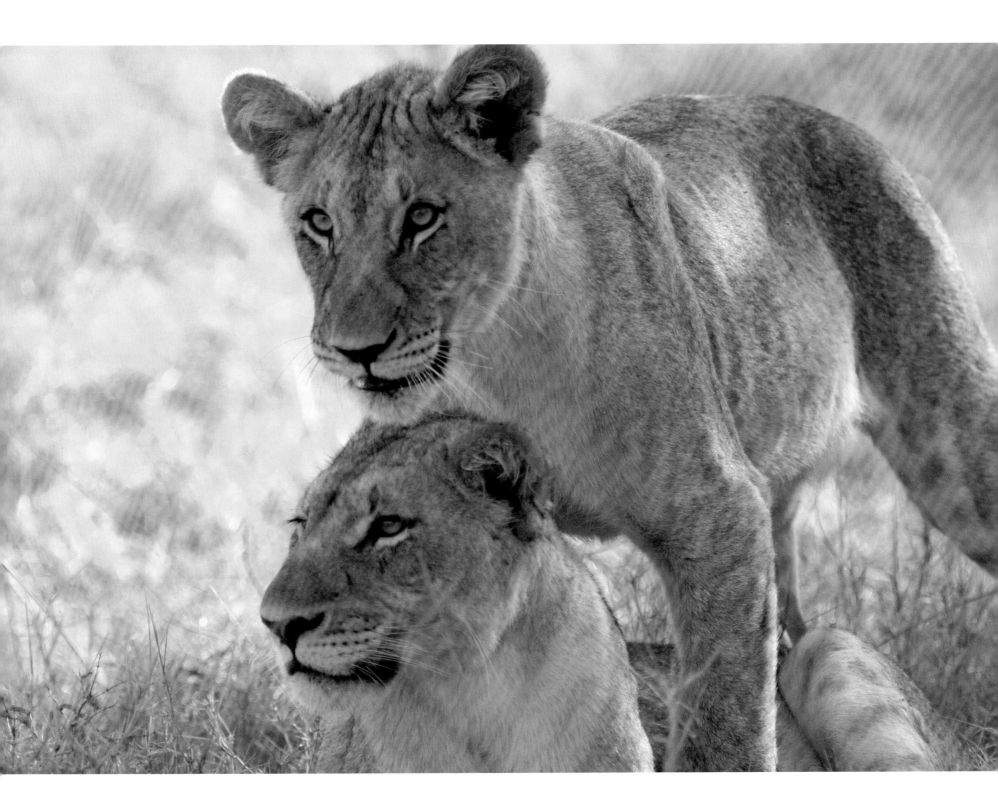

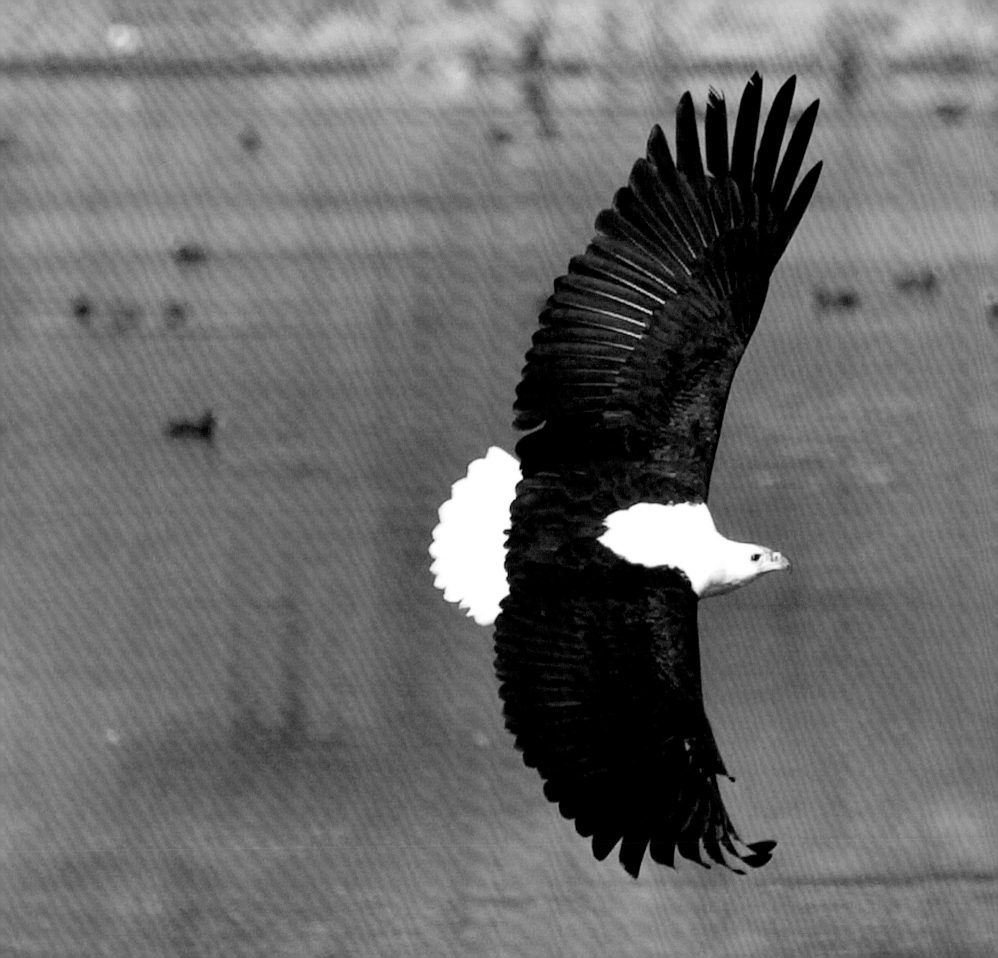

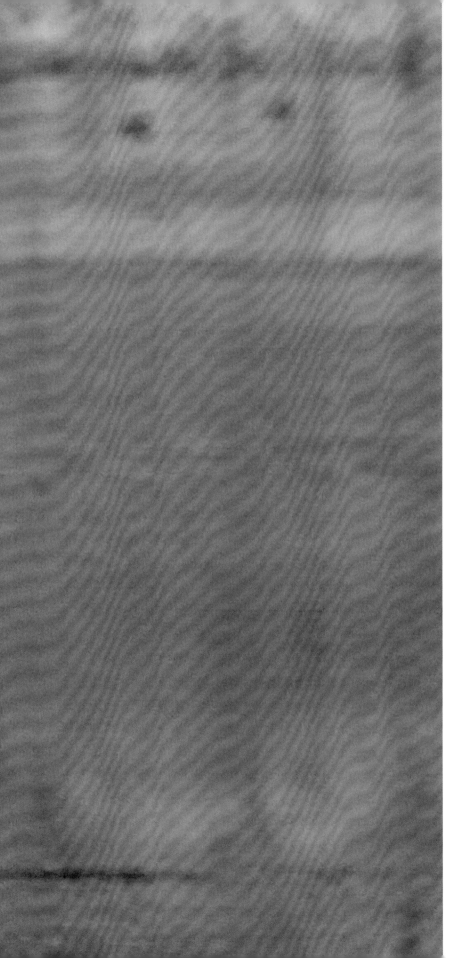

As I crossed the snow-covered plateau to stand with my fellow climbers for a victory photograph, I knew something of my self was being left behind. A part of me would always be in the thin air. I also realized how my choice of ascent had powerfully affected how I experienced the summit. With its gravel and open vista toward the plains below, the alternate approach I described would not allow a traveler to find his own way. It seemed to conceal the effort of the individual, obscuring footsteps in a path of rubble, and left little of the mountain's majesty to touch. My travelers and I had "cut a path" that would never be repeated. I was reminded of a quotation I kept on my desk during the many years of my recovery: "And if every way is closed before you, the secret one will show a secret path no other eyes have seen" (Rumi). I understood, as with all roads traveled in life, our choice of journey determines the summit we experience.

This trek released my own judgment of a broken body, which I'd held after nearly a decade of hamstring pain and fatigue. I may always have to watch my exertion and limit activities that cause discomfort, but now I understand that I can pace myself. When the symptoms of fatigue appear, I have the choice to accept rest and allow muscles to recover. In my own way and in my own time, I will reach the summit. I stand taller.

—Dana

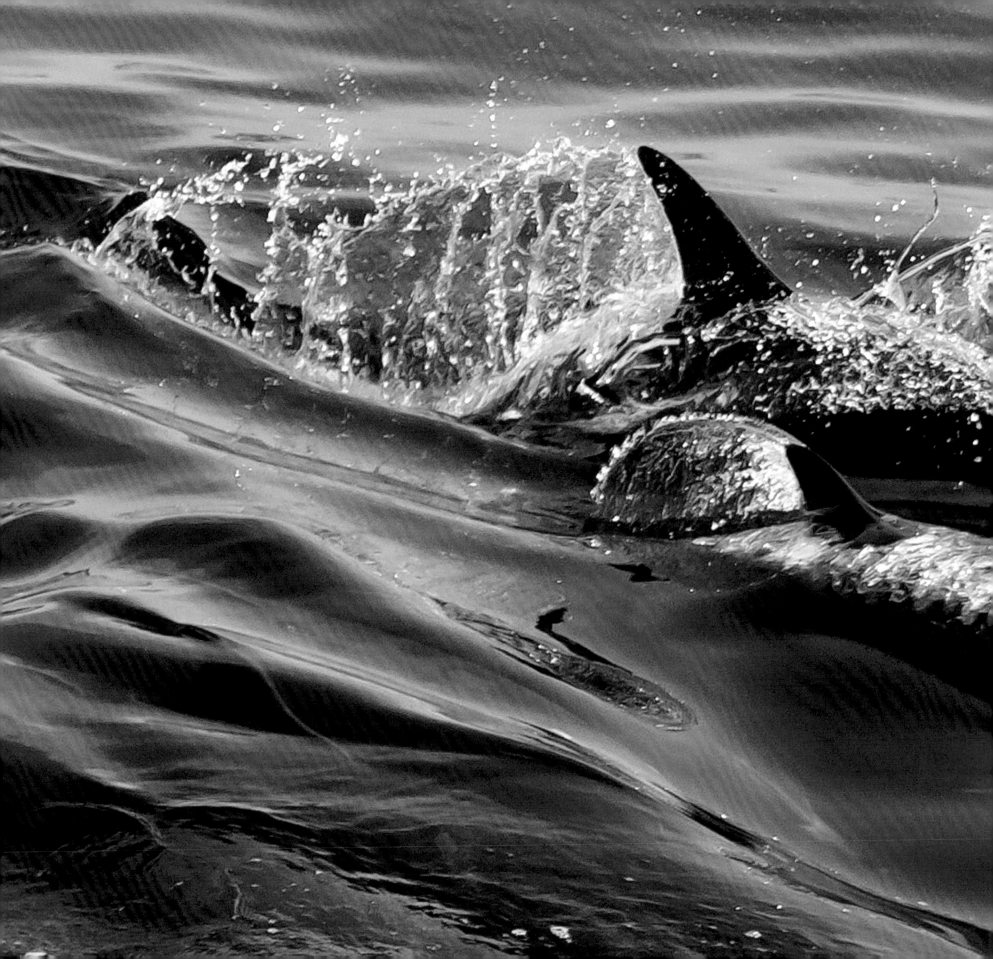

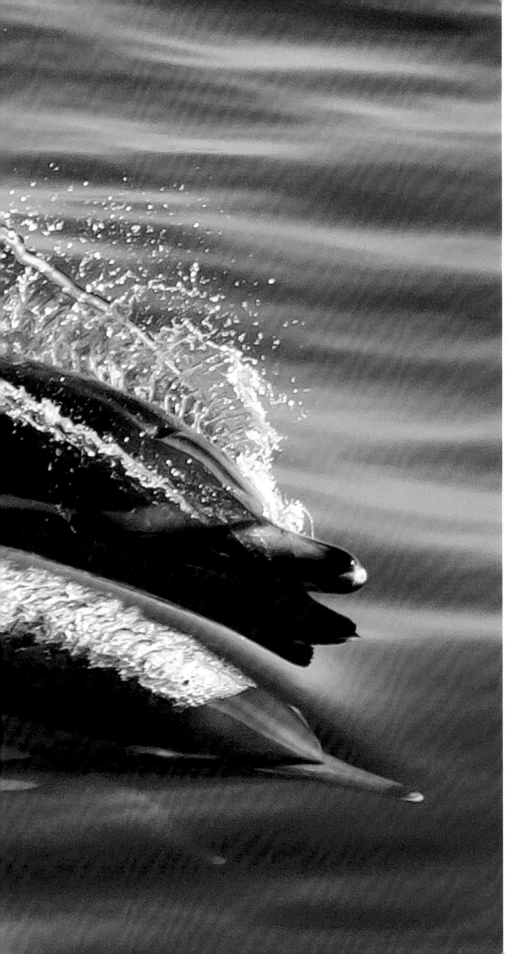

The Magic Sea
Ventura, California

We were gifted with a calm sea. Usually whitecaps and large swells are here between Ventura and the Channel Islands, but today it is as smooth as a lake. The Channel Islands are a chain of eight islands located in the Pacific Ocean, off the coast of Southern California. Earlier in my life, my father and brothers went fishing in this area, preferring an area off one of the islands in particular for bass and sometimes salmon. The few times I went along, the sea was very rough. Our trip to watch whales and dolphins may now be blessed with no seasickness.

We are barely out of the harbor when I hear exclamations of excitement. There they are, dozens of dolphins playing in our wake. They dance beside us, in and out of the water. Their smiling faces are so humanlike, pleasing the viewer. In fact, are they smiling? They appear delighted with our boat and with us, exhilarated by our screams as we run about for a better view. This pod is huge, maybe hundreds, everywhere around us. And we're still so close to land. What did we do to deserve this magnificence? I believe divine intervention has brought this perfection. The sea is still, calm, almost glassy, and all these wonderful creatures are jumping out of the water for a glimpse of us.

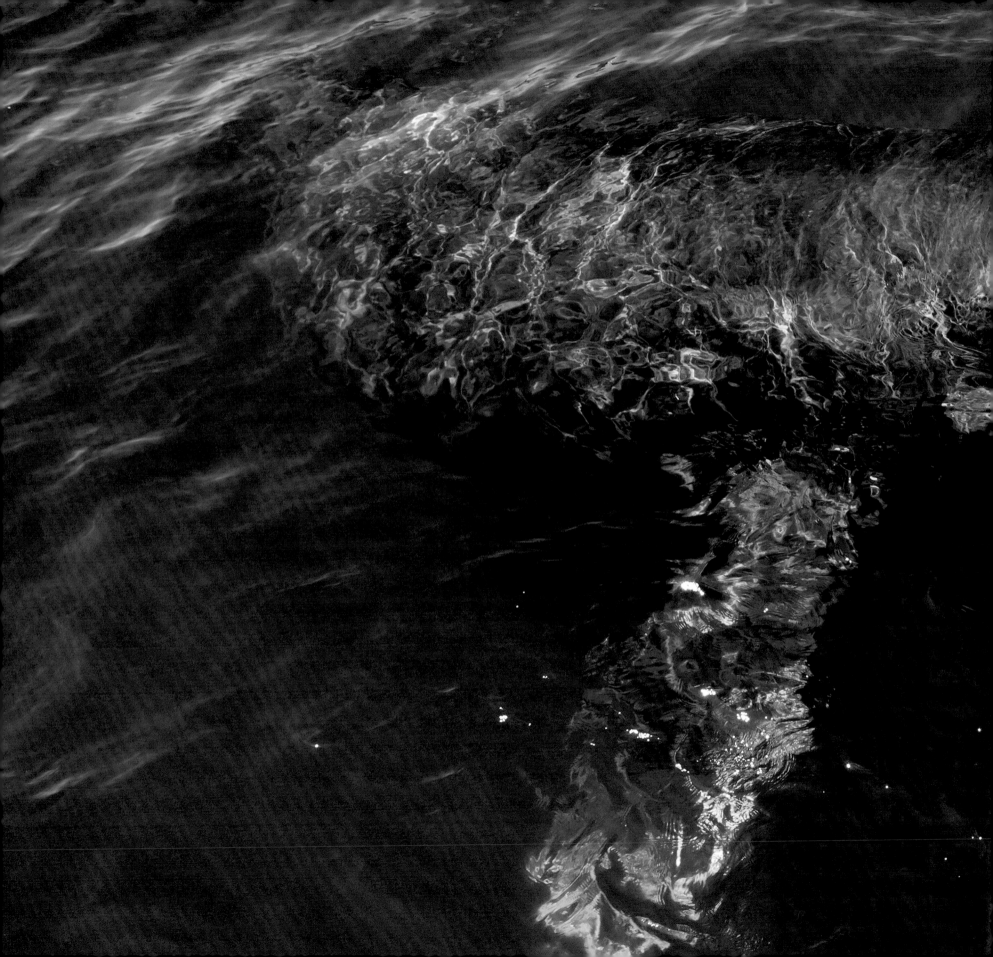

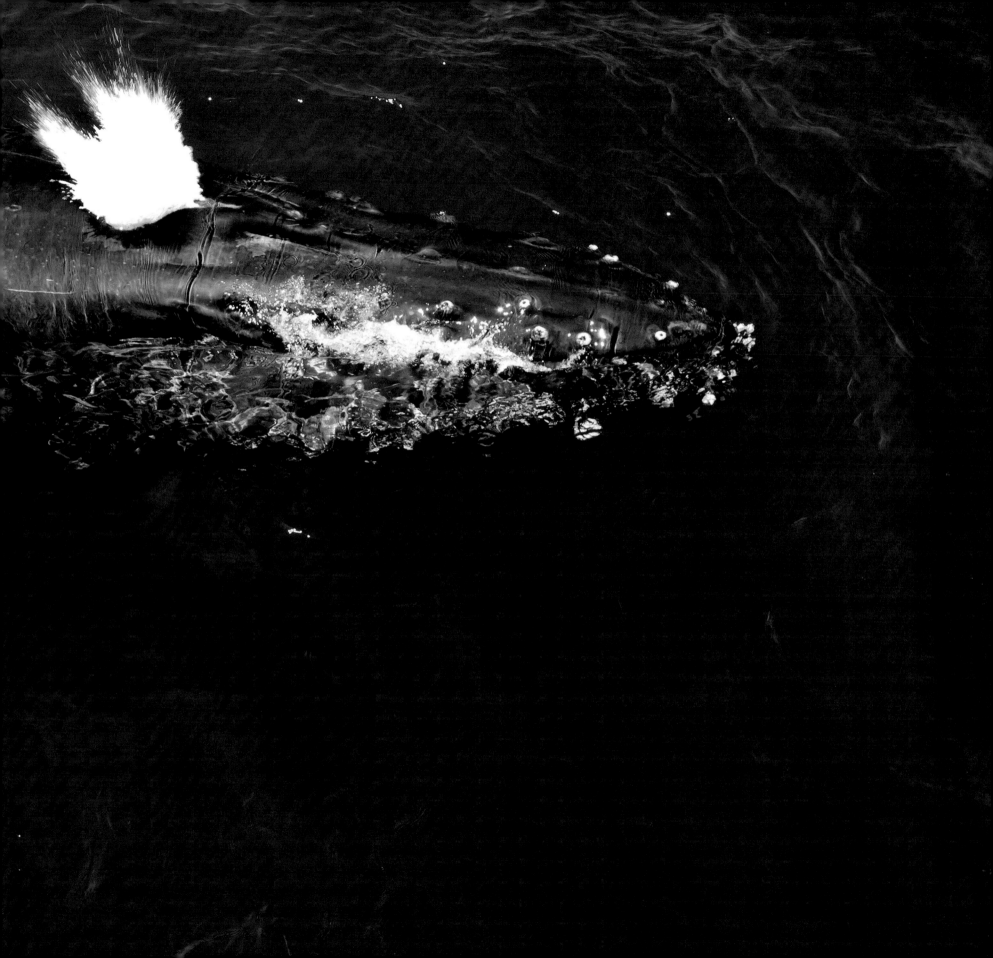

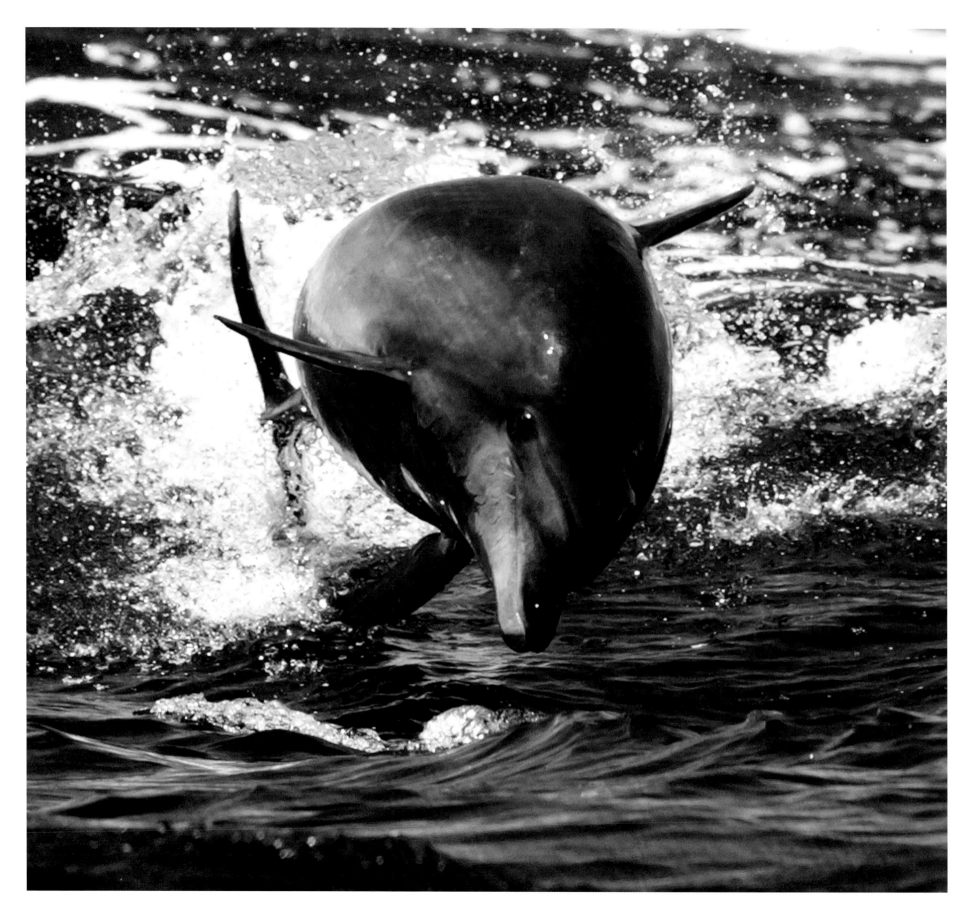

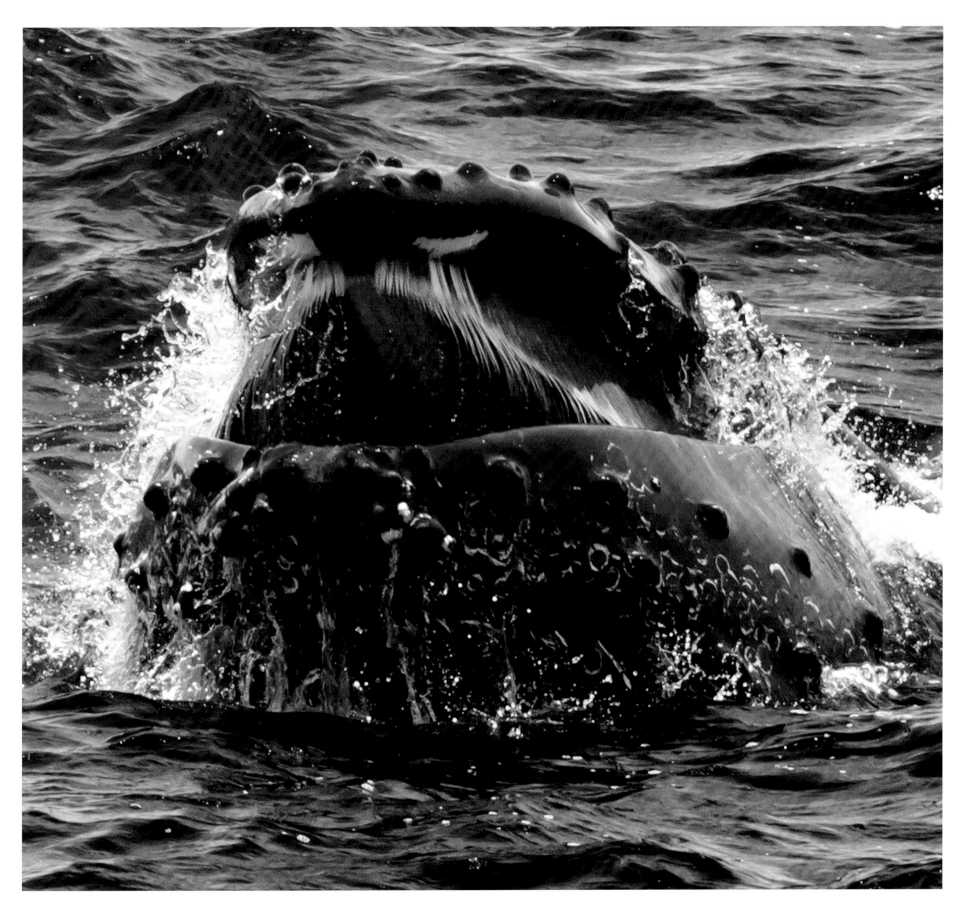

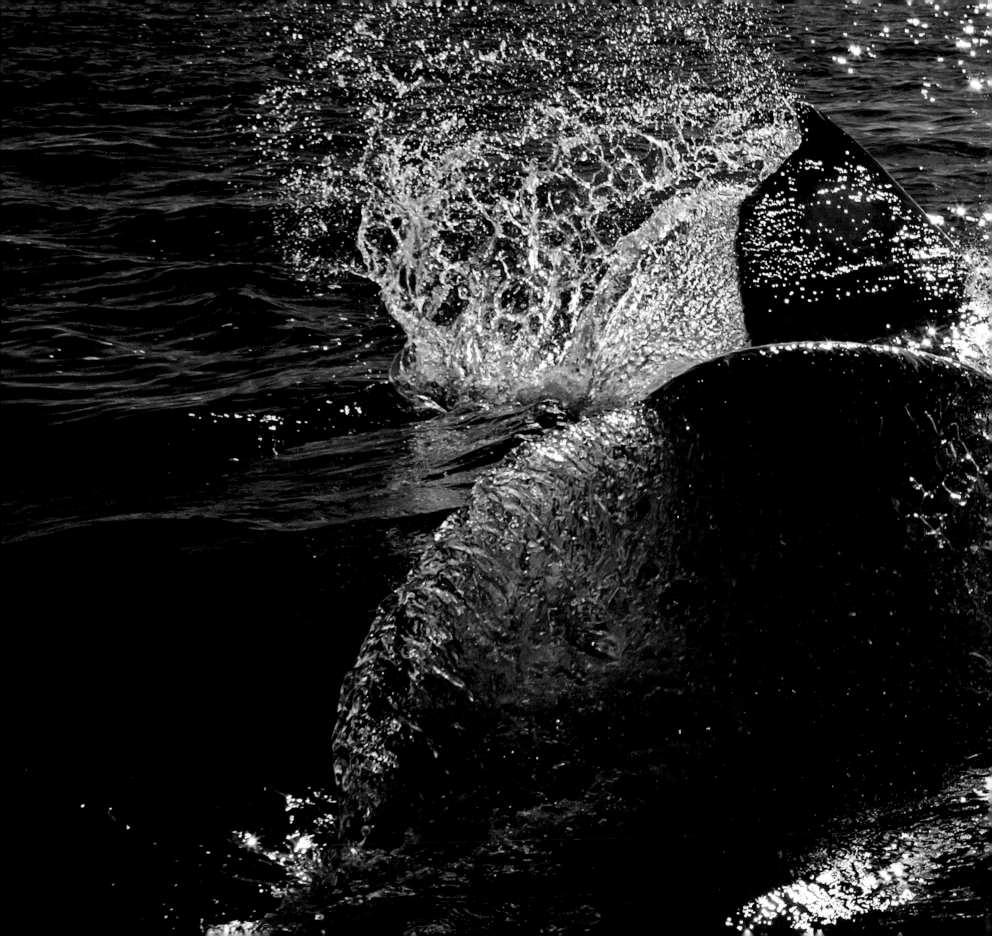

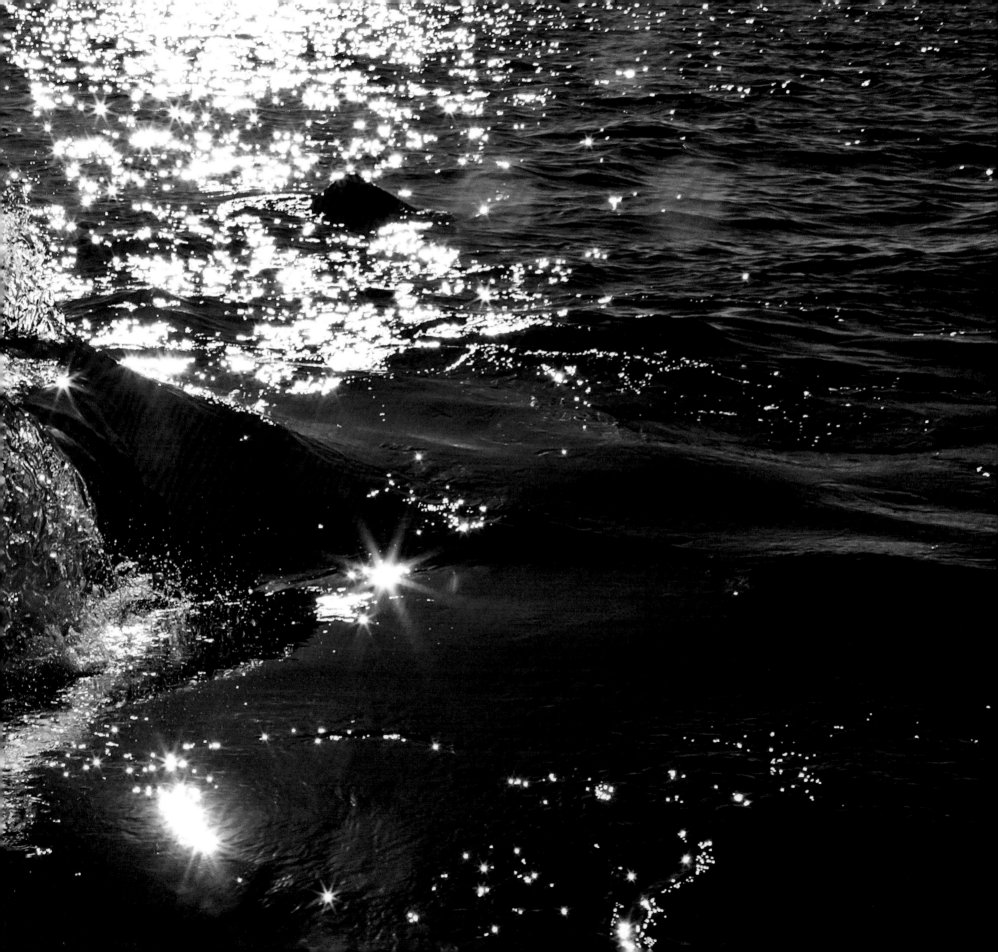

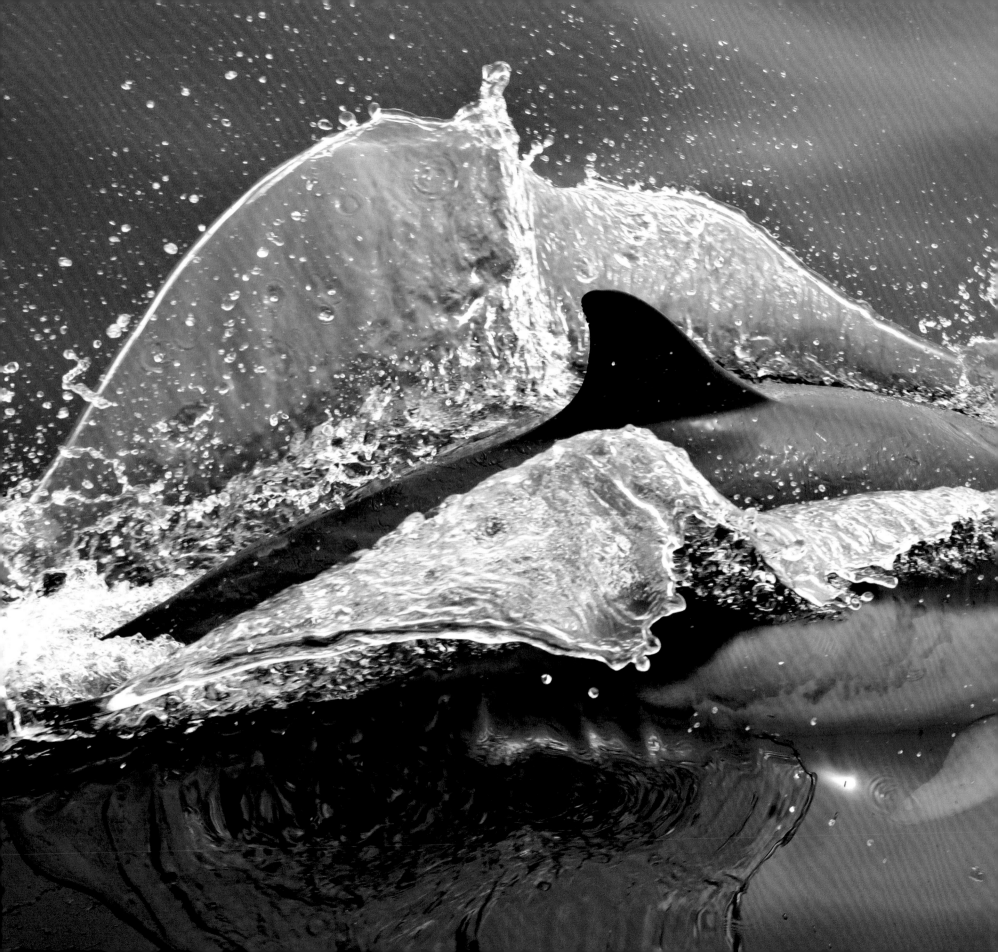

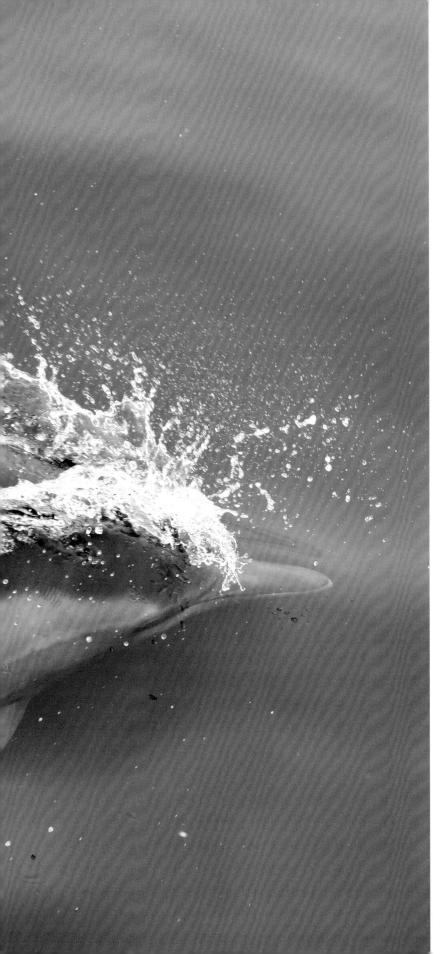

I wonder what these animals are here to teach me. I remember the lightness of my body in the water, but never the joyousness they seem to have. I could never end the chattering of my mind, endless planning and worrying, thoughts of my friends and the incessant critique of my own swim stroke. I could never silence the self-analysis. The dolphins are teaching me to let go, to let go of all those mental ways.

When I imagine my body moving so seamlessly in the sea, I feel an end to concerns about my physical limitations. The joy of those dolphins is clear to me now. But I am not to dwell with these fantasies for long, as I've come for photography. Tim, my teacher, is already shooting away. Despite the calm sea, the boat jerks some, and the dolphins move so fast. I can't find the stability to focus, and using a tripod on this crowded boat is out of the question. I must trust my nonvibration lens and just start, hoping that in editing, I'll find that, once or twice, I captured these moments.

Things change in the sea, and the whales appear. The grand beasts of the sea are breaching and twisting. Why they raise themselves out of the water gets many explanations from the experts, but the fact that they are so close to our boat is of greater interest by far. They understand their bodies and don't mistakenly fall back upon us, don't even touch the sides of our vessel. I feel again that I'm in a moment of grace, being so close to these huge creatures. They take my breath away.

–Karen

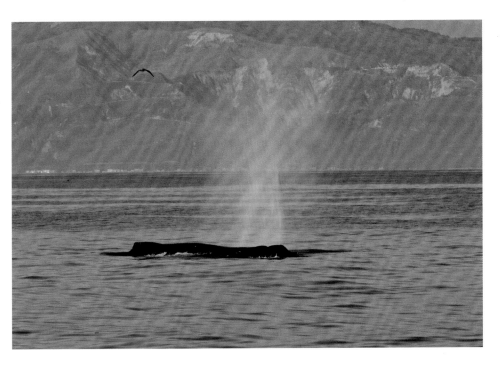

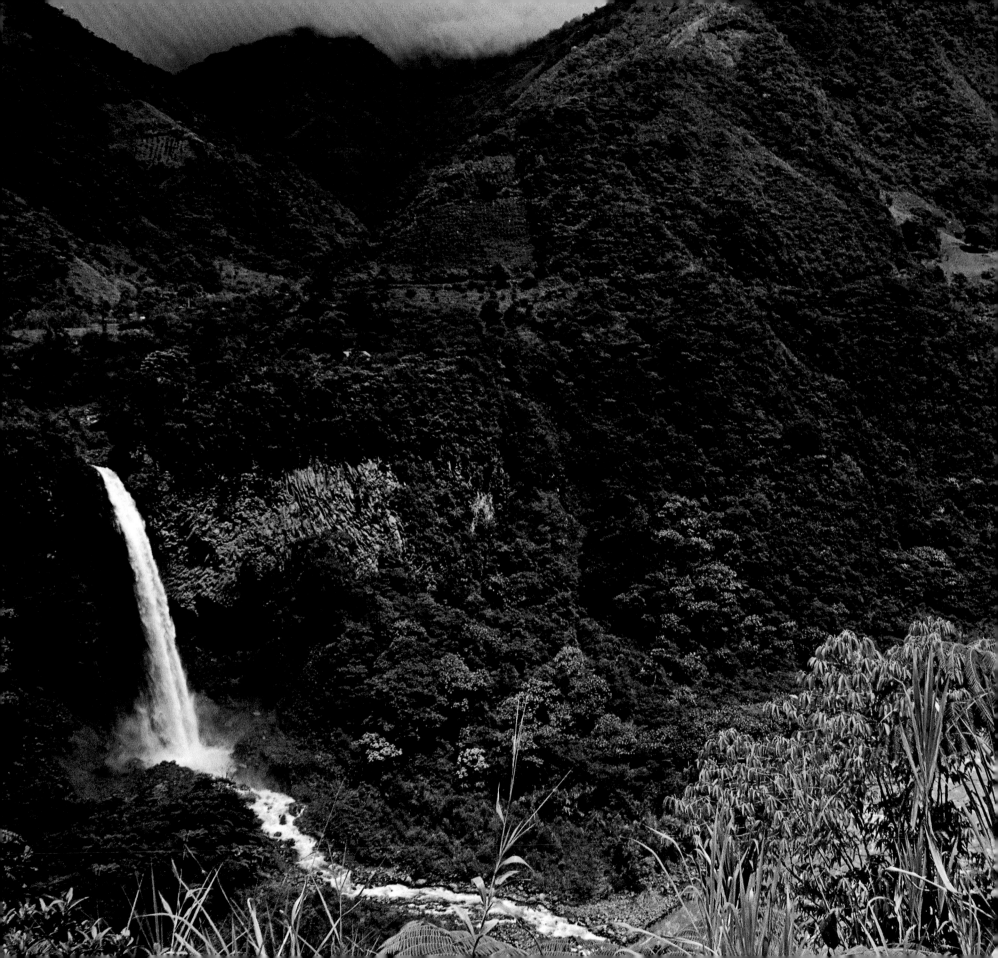

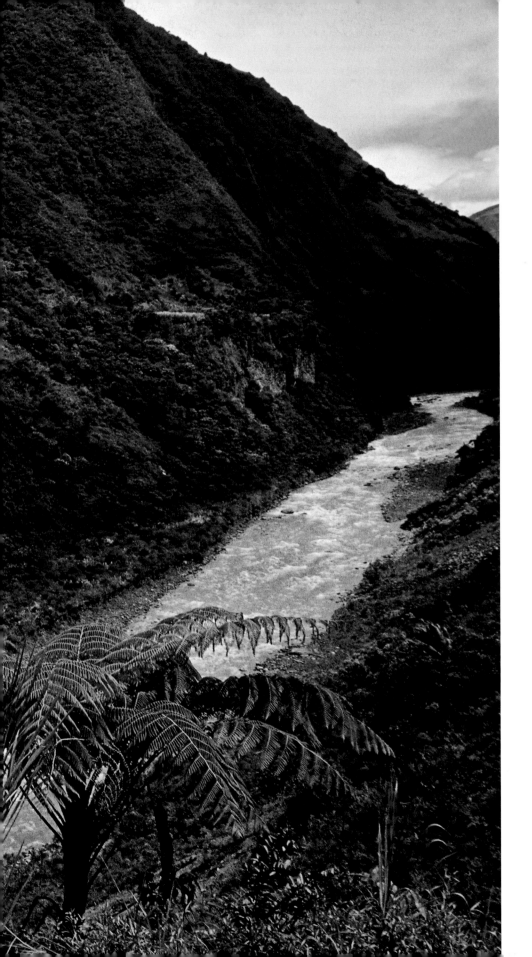

Conclusion

Decades of research have introduced many treatment options; however, both Lyme and MS fall within the "incurable" realm. Once diagnosed, one sees the future as an ever-changing variable, and decision making is shortened to the immediate. We reached for helping hands, which often meant searching out a new, sometimes esoteric, book. There were many stories, from many cultures, written by contemporary authors and writers from the past. We yearned for answers, as well as trustworthy guides. One might say we hoped to weave medicine and spirituality, to find understanding and acceptance. Each story deepened the integration of body, mind, and spirit.

Healing is a journey. We were blessed with opportunities to walk in new places. From public garden to mountain summit, we planted our feet in the earth and followed our heart's path. May this book, like the many that helped us, give you hope—the hope to find your way, and the quiet compassion to listen to your body's wisdom.

Thomas Eckert

Dana Simpson

Believe that a further shore
is reachable from here.
Believe in miracles
and cures and healing wells.

—Seamus Heaney, *The Cure at Troy* (1990)

Front cover
Raven, Scorpion Canyon, Santa Cruz Island, Channel Islands National Park, California

Back cover
Colorado Columbine, Ptarmagine Loop Trail, Vail Mountain, Colorado

Front matter
1) Raven
2/3) Scorpion Canyon, Santa Cruz Island, Channel Islands National Park, California
5) Meditation Mount, Ojai, California
6/7) Fishing boat, Regional Nature Park of the Camargue, France

Introduction
8/9) Milford Sound near Homer Tunnel, Fiordland National Park, New Zealand

Shear Harmony
10) Mirror Lake, Milford Sound Road
12/13) Sunrise, Lake Rotorua
14) Waimakariri River Valley, Authur's Pass
15) Milford Sound, Fiordland National Park
16/17) Lake Matheson with Mount Cook in background
18) Limestone caves, Oparara River Reserve
19) Falls River, Abel Tasman National Park
20 top) Sheep near Queenstown
20 bottom) Sheep shearing, Waimakariri River Valley
21) Milford Sound Road

Sand and Soil
22) Hendry's Beach
24) Midden site, San Miguel Island, Channel Islands National Park
25) Peregrine falcon
26/27) Mesa Lane Beach / Thousand Steps Beach
28/29) Torrey Pine Forest, Santa Rosa Island, Channel Islands National Park
30) Alice Keck Park Memorial Gardens
31 left) Alice Keck Park Memorial Gardens
31 right) Alice Keck Park Memorial Gardens
32/33) Hendry's Beach

Reaching Out
34/35) Ptarmigan Loop Trail, Vail Mountain
36) Booth Creek Falls, White River National Forest
37) Booth Creek Falls, White River National Forest
38/39) Grand Escape Trail, Vail Mountain
40) Betty Ford Alpine Gardens
41) White River National Forest
42) Betty Ford Alpine Gardens
43) Colorado Columbine

Diagnosis to Freedom
44) View of Ojai Valley from Meditation Mount
45) American bald eagle
46) Oak tree
47 top) Matilija poppy
47 bottom) Flower stand
48/49) Lake Casitas
50) Orange groves
51) Topa Topa bluffs from Ojai Valley
52) Creek Road
53) Shelf Road waterfall

Surfacing
54) Shearwater, Santa Barbara Channel
56/57) Goleta pier
58) Beach at Coal Oil Point
59) Oak tree and clouds
60) Springtime wildflowers, San Rafael Wilderness
61) Springtime wildflowers near Gorman
62) Goleta swimming pool

The Raven's Call
64) Scorpion Canyon, Santa Cruz Island, Channel Islands National Park
67) Delphine's Grove, Santa Cruz Island, Channel Islands National Park

The Raven's Call (continued)
68) Sunrise, Montañon Ridge, Santa Cruz Island, Channel Islands National Park
70/71) San Miguel Island, Channel Islands National Park
72) Santa Cruz Island, Channel Islands National Park
74/75) South Fork Eel River, Humboldt Redwoods State Park
76) James Irvine Trail, Prairie Creek Redwoods National and State Park
77) Redwoods National Park

Being Guided
78) Emerald Pools Nature Trail
80 left) East Rim Trail
81) Virgin River
82/83) Moon setting, Towers of the Virgin
84) Echo Canyon
85) Antelope Canyon
86) Swallowtail butterfly
87) Emerald Pools Nature Trail

Cloud Forest
88) Tungurahua Volcano
89) Hummingbird, Bellavista Cloud Forest Reserve
90/91) Bellavista Cloud Forest Reserve
92/93) Flora, Bellavista Cloud Forest Reserve
94/95) Bellavista Cloud Forest Reserve
96) Local women near Tungurahua Volcano
97) Market at Otavalo

Black Bulls, White Horses
98) Greater flamingos, Regional Nature Park of the Camargue
99) Greater flamingos courtship, Regional Nature Park of the Camargue
100) Camargue bull, Regional Nature Park of the Camargue
101) Camargue horses, Regional Nature Park of the Camargue
102/103) Hot air ballooning, Chalon-sur-Saône
104) Salin de Badon marsh, Regional Nature Park of the Camargue
105) Little egret, Regional Nature Park of the Camargue
106) Local bullfight

Birdsong and Silence
108) Lago Pehoe and the Paine massif, Torres del Paine National Park
109) Curious guanacos, Torres del Paine National Park
110 left) Torres del Paine, Torres del Paine National Park
110 right) Mirador las Torres, Torres del Paine National Park
111) Cuernos del Paine, Torres del Paine National Park
112/113) Salto Grande, Torres del Paine National Park
114) Magellanic penguins, Isla Magdalena Natural Monument
115) Icebergs, Lago Grey, Torres del Paine National Park
116/117) Paso los Cuernos, Torres del Paine National Park
118) Trail riding, Torres del Paine National Park

Standing Taller
120) Burchell's zebras
122) Male lion
123) Cheetah
124/125) Blue wildebeest (gnu)
126) Hippopotamus
127) African elephant cow and calf
128) Long-crested eagle
129) Lion cubs
130) African fish eagle

The Magic Sea
132) Common dolphins
134/135) Humpback whale
136) Bottlenose dolphin
137) Humpback whale lunge feeding
138/139) Gray whale
140) Common dolphin
141) Humpback whales

Conclusion
142) Cascada Mondo de la Novia, Ecuador